The Sleeping Pill

Other Books by Ernest Hartmann

The Biology of Dreaming, 1967

Adolescents in a Mental Hospital,
   with B. Glasser, M. Greenblatt,
   M. Solomon, and D. Levinson, 1968

Sleep and Dreaming, 1970

The Functions of Sleep, 1973

THE
SLEEPING PILL

ERNEST HARTMANN, M.D.

NEW HAVEN AND LONDON   YALE UNIVERSITY PRESS   1978

Designed by Sally Harris
and set in VIP Caledonia type.
Printed in the United States of America by
Vail-Ballou Press, Binghamton, New York.

Published in Great Britain, Europe, Africa, and
Asia (except Japan) by Yale University Press,
Ltd., London. Distributed in Australia and New
Zealand by Book & Film Services, Artarmon,
N.S.W., Australia; and in Japan by Harper &
Row, Publishers, Tokyo Office.

Library of Congress Cataloging in Publication Data

Hartmann, Ernest.
  The sleeping pill.

  Includes bibliographical references and index.
  1. Hypnotics. 2. Insomnia. I. Title. [DNLM: 1. Hypnotics and sedatives–Therapeutic use. 2. Insomnia–Drug therapy. QV85 H333s]
RM325.H37   615'.782   78-6205
ISBN 0-300-02248-4

Contents

Figures

Tables

Acknowledgments

This is my work, and I must take full responsibility and blame for it. However, a large number of persons have been of immense help to me. In fact, as soon as I begin to think about it, my debt to others is so great that I despair of mentioning them all. Those I do mention below made contributions, probably far greater than they believe, and I am deeply grateful for their help.

Larry Hartmann and Myron Sharaf read portions of the manuscript and made extremely useful suggestions which I have incorporated into the chapter on the psychodynamics of the sleeping pill. Eva Hartmann, Cheryl Spinweber, Molly Oldfield, Diane Russ, and Eric Sorrin all read the manuscript, or large portions of it, and contributed and made many useful suggestions and corrections. Martha Monahan and Cynthia Angel had an important part in the actual writing of chapter 2, and both also read and made suggestions on the rest of the text. Maureen Muchowski patiently and perfectly typed and retyped many versions of this work, and often had to deal with my very difficult handwriting and dictation.

I would also like to express my thanks to my many collaborators in the sleep research projects which laid a foundation for great portions of this book. James Cravens, Cheryl Spinweber, Quentin Regestein, Richard Elion, Val Pochay, Maressa Orzack, Roland Branconnier, George Zwilling, and Warren Stern have all been important collaborators. I am indebted to Drs. Jonathan Cole and Milton Greenblatt, who have been my teachers, catalysts, and instigators of research, as well as my friends, while they directed the institutions in which my work was performed.

Research, unfortunately, always requires money, and I am grateful to a number of institutes and branches of the United States Department of Health, Education, and Welfare, as well as to several private corporations which made the research possible. Some of the research was greatly facilitated by the smooth functioning of the Sleep Research Foundation, and I would thus like to express special thanks to my friends—and sometimes critics—who are trustees of the foundation: Alan Lazerson, Myron Sharaf, George Vaillant, Leonard Solomon, and our lawyer, William Rollins.

Finally, my thanks to the Association for the Psychophysiological Study of Sleep, a society which has managed to combine high scientific standards with informality and friendship in such a way as to make sleep research basically an enjoyable undertaking.

1

Introduction

The first cry for relief from
pain and sleeplessness has been called the beginning of
medicine, and it is also the beginning of pharmacology. We
can picture an eternally recurring scene: the sufferer, his face
lined with pain, with sorrow, with sleeplessness, calls out—
and lo! relief appears. A well-dressed gentleman bearing a
diploma and a pill? A sorcerer with a steaming potion? A
demigod with an elixir? Or perhaps the cry is answered in
another way by the still more potent god or angel who grants
final relief from suffering, and the deepest sleep. Socrates,
with his final words, "I owe a cock to Asclepius," was repay-
ing the god of medicine for the hemlock that finally relieved
him of all suffering.

To a certain extent life *is* pain and sorrow. The path to
relief must be taken cautiously, for it is also the path to
death. It is not entirely surprising, then, that drugs which
relieve pain and sleeplessness are also drugs which bring
death. As we shall see, up to now the drugs used to produce
sleep have been nonspecific central nervous system depressants ("deadeners"): they are drugs which deaden wakefulness, pain and sorrow. And they do their job well, sometimes
too well.

In this book I first examine briefly the history of the sleeping pill from ancient Egypt and Greece to the present. Next,
currently available sleeping medications are listed, classified,
and discussed. I then attempt a statistical examination of certain questions such as who takes sleeping pills and who
prescribes them, what kinds, and how much (chap. 3).

It becomes obvious that we cannot go further in examining
the action of sleeping pills unless we understand something

1

about sleep. Chapter 4 reviews our current knowledge of sleep, including the ways it is being studied, its physiology and chemistry, and its possible functions. In chapter 5, I discuss and summarize all human sleep laboratory studies involving the effects of hypnotic drugs on sleep.

We may conclude that many, though perhaps not all, current sleeping pills do have some effect in inducing sleep. However, we begin to see that there are numerous problems: drugs do not maintain their effectiveness when used continuously; most drugs produce distortions in normal sleep patterns, both when they are being taken and after they have been discontinued; some also produce detrimental effects on waking behavior while they are being administered. Chapter 5 condenses a great deal of material, and it can be used as a source for references to other specific studies. The reader who is interested in methodology and a detailed description of specific drug studies can read the reports in Appendices A and B.

I then turn to a more careful consideration of insomnia: who has trouble sleeping and why, and which insomniacs may require sleeping pills. Chapter 6 presents a classification of insomnia, and a discussion of the treatment of insomnia within the limits of our current knowledge. The conclusion here is that insomnia is not an illness for which a sleeping pill is the cure. Rather, insomnia is a symptom, and there are a great many causes of insomnia. These causes require specific treatment for particular medical or psychiatric problems. Often, the most effective treatment does not involve medication at all, or if medication is required it may be an antidepressant, an antipsychotic, or a drug to treat a specific medical illness. Only a relatively small number of people actually require sleeping pills.

In chapter 7 I discuss the psychodynamics of the sleeping pill—in other words, why do so many people take sleeping pills and why do so many doctors prescribe them? Why does this occur even in situations where sleeping pills are not the best treatment? One of the most common forms of human interaction is the following: a person who labels himself as a sufferer, someone in need of help, goes to another person labeled doctor, or giver of help, to find relief from physical or mental suffering. For many complicated reasons, the complaint—or suffering—is often expressed in the words "I have trouble sleeping." Sleep is easily disrupted in many people and thus becomes a scapegoat, readily and conveniently seized upon. The response of the other person—the doctor—again for many different psychological reasons, is often to provide the patient with a potion or pill: the sleeping pill.

The risks and benefits associated with the use of sleeping pills are then summarized and discussed in chapter 8. Sleeping pills do work—they do produce sleep, or something closely resembling normal sleep—at least when first administered—but they are generally dangerous, easily abused, nonspecific central nervous system depressants; their effects last longer than we would like, and they have disturbing interactions with other medications. The conclusion is drawn that in an overall sense the risks of sleeping pills, as they are actually used, appear to outweigh the benefits.

In my view, the dangers and problems associated with these substances (see chap. 8) stem from the fact that their actions bear no relationship to the normal physiology or chemistry of sleep. They are simply nonspecific central nervous system depressants. If one opens a pharmacology textbook to the chapter on *hypnotics* (sleeping pills), one finds a list of medications including barbiturates, nonbarbiturates, and so on. Then, turning a few pages, one finds many of these same substances—especially the barbiturates—also listed in the chapter on *anesthetics*. Thus, the same chemical substances produce sleep at one dose and anesthesia at another (higher) dose. If the textbook should happen to include a chapter on poisons or agents that produce coma and death, the same substances will appear again.

I discuss in chapters 9 and 10 three different lines of research that could lead to a more rational and safer sleeping pill—one whose action is related to the known chemistry of sleep. One possibility involves research on endogenous brain peptides that may play a role in mechanisms underlying pain and sleep. Another relates to drugs which block or alter the activity of brain catecholamines. Third (chap. 10), I discuss in more detail a line of investigation I have already been pursuing for some years: studies of the natural amino acid l-tryptophan, a precursor of brain serotonin. Results demonstrating the sleep-inducing effects of l-tryptophan in animals and humans are presented.

The final chapter reviews what I have discussed about insomnia, its treatment, and past, present, and future sleeping pills. It also includes suggestions for present action and future research.

To my scientific colleagues in the field, I must state that, while I have done a great deal of research in the area of sleep, this book is not a report on a piece of research, though it includes in the appendices several specific laboratory studies. This is, rather, a series of essays derived from sleep research and is obviously full of my own formulations and conclusions. The conclusions are open to criticism and debate and will, I hope, inspire a good deal of both.

A few years ago I wrote a book entitled *The Functions of Sleep* which attempted to outline a complete theory about the functional role of sleep. The present work is not a theory in that sense. Nor is this book a complete encyclopedia or compendium of sleeping pills—their basic pharmacology, pharmacodynamics, and so on. I present a great many facts about hypnotic medications or sleeping pills and review a number of laboratory studies that have evaluated them. I use these facts as a background for presenting some views about what is required in the development of sleeping pills, about the nature, treatment (and mistreatment) of insomnia, and about the limited place I believe sleeping pills have in its treatment. I point out that, so far, our methods of developing sleeping pills have resulted simply in ever more nonspecific central nervous system depressants and poisons. I conclude that for sleeping pills as a class the risks outweigh the benefits. All this obviously calls for change, and I discuss some possibilities.

Except in the chapters and appendices presenting actual sleep research work, I have not tried to be complete in terms of bibliographical references for each chapter. Since several thousand articles and reports dealing with sleeping pills and the pharmacology of sleep have been published in the last ten years alone, completeness would be impossible in a work of this size. I have, in many cases, referred to other books and reviews that I felt would be most helpful to a reader not already familiar with the field. I have at times referred to specific research articles when they are especially relevant to a particular point, but I have not attempted to cite every report that deserves credit for a given point. I believe my approach will be useful to most readers, but it does result in some unevenness in references; I hope this will not be too disconcerting to my colleagues who are accustomed to greater uniformity.

The terms *sleeping pill* and *hypnotic medication* are synonymous and are here used interchangeably. I tend to prefer the simpler term *sleeping pill* since it somewhat demystifies these substances. The longer, more "scientific" term makes it sound as though a group of scientists, basing their work on the biology of sleep and insomnia, had carefully developed these drugs in terms of their relation to sleep and had officially pronounced them "hypnotic medication." This, as we shall see, is by no means the case.

2

Sleeping Pills, Past
and Present

A Brief History of the
Sleeping Pill

The ability to achieve sleep
has always been important and has at times been considered
sacred. One of the less powerful deities in the Greek pantheon,
but one consistently worshipped, was Hypnos the god of sleep,
who swept over land and sea bringing sleep to men and gods
alike. He is usually represented bearing a poppy stalk and a
horn from which he drops slumber upon those he visits
(figure 2.1). Indeed, the juice of the poppy was perhaps the
first "sleeping pill," and it is not an exaggeration to say that
the poppy (especially its derivatives, morphine and heroin)
has been and still is worshipped almost as a god. Products of
the poppy were used by the Romans, the Greeks, and perhaps
the Egyptians for several centuries before Christ. In the first
century A.D., Scribonius Largus, in *De Compositione Medi-
camentorum,* had already described the preparation of relatively pure opium from the juice of the poppy.

The efficacy of the poppy and its juices is attested to in
almost every ancient medical text, including those of Aretaeus
of Cappadocia, Diascorides, Lucian, and Celsus. There is apparently no mention of the poppy in the extant works of
Hippocrates, but he was known as a sort of drug nihilist who
had little faith in any of the medications then available.

The mandrake tree, or mandragora, was also clearly recognized by Greek and Roman physicians as possessing hypnotic
and narcotic properties. In 300 B.C., the Greek physician
Theophrastus prescribed mandrake for sleeplessness, though

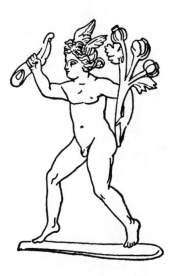

FIGURE 2.1   *Hypnos*

admittedly he also recommended it for wounds, gout, and
use in love potions. Hyoscyamus, a common plant also referred
to as henbane and swinebean, was widely prescribed as a
hypnotic by ancient Greek physicians. The milk of common
lettuce was frequently prescribed to induce sleep. Galen
particularly recommended a prescription for sleep consisting
of the bark of mandragora, the seed of black henbane, and
opium—all mixed with the juice of lettuce: this potion was
either taken internally or was rubbed into the temples. In
addition, mulberry and hellebore were frequently used. Although hellebore was chiefly used as a purgative in the
ancient world, Theophrastus noted its sedative properties as
well. Figure 2.2 illustrates some of these early herbal "sleeping pills."

Very similar, plant-derived substances were apparently used

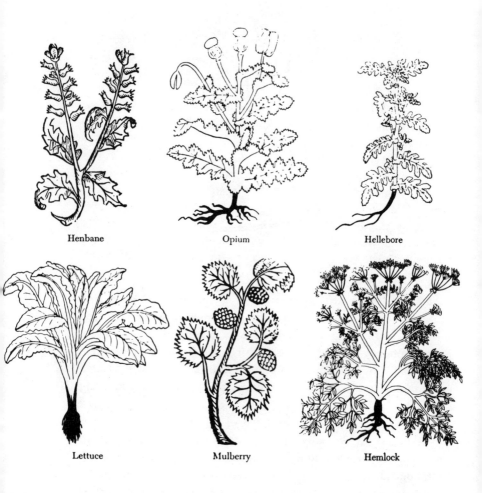

Henbane

Opium

Hellebore

Lettuce

Mulberry

Hemlock

FIGURE 2.2 Early Herbal "Sleeping Pills"

by physicians of the Middle East. The *Arabian Nights* contains an account of the use of a soporific:

Presently he filled a cresset with firewood on which he strewed powdered henbane and, lighting it, went around about the tent with it till the smoke entered the nostrils of the guards and they fell asleep, drowned by the drug.

Avicenna, the famous Arabian physician, in his *Canon of Medicine* recommends opium, henbane, and mandrake for producing sleep.

In the Middle Ages and the Renaissance basically the same ingredients were used, in different mixtures and sometimes combined with alcohol. The most famous hypnotic of the Middle Ages was called "spongia somnifera." This was a sponge steeped in wine and a mixture of opium, lettuce, hemlock, hyoscyamus, mulberry juice, mandragora, and ivy; this was used both to induce sleep and as an anesthetic. The various mixtures of this time, with some variations in ingredients, were widely available in apothecary shops and on medicine shelves at home, and were generally referred to as "drowsy syrups."

Shakespeare, in *Othello*, refers to the same familiar substances:

> Not poppy nor mandragora,
> Nor all the drowsy syrups of the world,
> Shall ever medicine thee to that sweet sleep
> Which thou hadst yesterday.*

Of course, certain social relaxants, especially alcohol and to some extent marijuana and hashish, have at times over the centuries been used as sleeping pills.

The same herbs and plants referred to above continued to be the most widely employed hypnotics through the end of the nineteenth century, and some are still used in many parts of the world today. From our present vantage point we sometimes find it easy to criticize past practices in medicine: no

---

* And Shakespeare makes the same point I make later (chap. 6): one cannot ignore the cause of an insomnia and simply treat it with a sleeping pill.

placebo-controlled, double-blind studies were done then; there was no uniformity in measurement of dosage, and so on. Often we conclude that until the last century or so medicine was chiefly magic and medication chiefly placebo—made to work, if it worked at all, by power of suggestion of the physician. It is noteworthy that in the case of the sleeping pill such criticism is not justified: the most widely used ancient herbs and potions have all turned out to contain chemicals which do indeed produce sedation and sleep.

Only recently have pharmacological techniques revealed the active ingredients in these plants, and it has been shown that the various sleeping medications contained a relatively small number of chemical alkaloids which produce sleep. The poppy, of course, contains the opium alkaloids, especially morphine and codeine. Mandragora and most of the others contain combinations of hyoscine, atropine, and scopolamine. These substances are still employed in currently used chemical hypnotics. In fact morphine is occasionally used to produce sleep when a powerful drug is required, and scopolamine, in small quantities, is still found in some over-the-counter sleeping medications.

In 1805 Frederick Seturner synthesized an active substance from crude extract of opium, found that it readily produced sleep in dogs, and named it "morphine" after the god of sleep and dreams, Morpheus (the Roman counterpart to Hypnos). In 1864, H. Behrend reported the use of potassium bromide as a treatment for insomnia and nervous excitement. Since then, a large number of pure chemicals of different classes have been introduced as hypnotic agents; these will be discussed in the following section.

SLEEPING PILLS IN
CURRENT USE

The hypnotics that were introduced to medicine in the nineteenth and early twentieth centuries and their derivatives are still in common use today. New hypnotics are being added almost yearly. This section briefly reviews the major hypnotic drugs in current use. A review of the effects of hypnotics on laboratory-recorded sleep appears in chapter 7.

Bromides The bromides were originally introduced into medicine in 1857 by Sir Charles Locock, in his treatment of epilepsy. An article published in 1864 indicated that these substances were also useful in treating insomnia and nervous excitement. Bromides enjoyed worldwide popularity in the late nineteenth and early twentieth centuries; they were chiefly used as anticonvulsants and sedatives, and occasionally as sleeping pills too. Unfortunately, the therapeutic index for the bromides is very low—in other words, the toxic dose is not much higher than the effective dose; therefore the bromides are quite dangerous substances. Any of the bromide salts (sodium bromide, potassium bromide, ammonium bromide, etc.) are effective as central nervous system depressants, but the required dosage is in the range of 3–5 grams per day. The mechanism of action involves the actual replacement of the chloride ion by the bromide ion in the central nervous system and other tissues.

Recognition of the toxicity of the bromides and discovery of less toxic, more efficacious agents have resulted in their infrequent use today.

Chloral Hydrate and
Related Compounds The oldest of the hypnotic agents, chloral hydrate, is a very simple chemical compound (fig. 2.3). It was first synthesized in 1832 by Liebig and came into general use as a hypnotic late in the nineteenth century. The use of chloral derivatives waned when the more powerful barbiturates were introduced. However, in the last twenty to thirty years chloral hydrate has once again become popular; it is frequently prescribed for all types of patients, including the medically ill and the elderly. Chloral hydrate has been

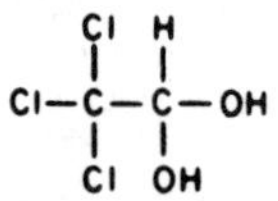

Chloral Hydrate 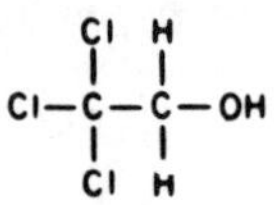   Trichloroethanol

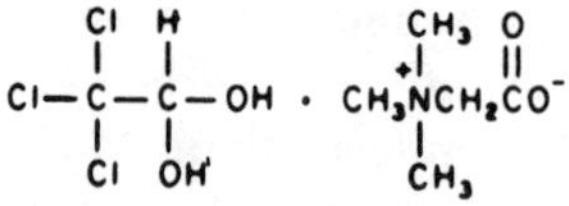

Chloral Betaine 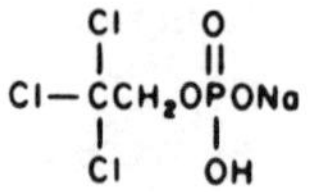   Triclofos Sodium

FIGURE 2.3   Chloral Hydrate and Its Derivatives

often used for patients unable to tolerate barbiturate medication.

The exact mechanism of action of chloral hydrate is unknown. In the body, chloral hydrate is rapidly reduced to trichloroethanol (fig. 2.3), which itself also has hypnotic properties. Thus, it is probable that the central depressant effects of chloral hydrate are actually due to the formation of trichloroethanol. Both substances clearly act as depressants of the central nervous system, and it is believed that their action is chiefly on the cerebral hemispheres.

Chloral hydrate is absorbed very rapidly and sleep usually begins within thirty minutes of administration. With therapeutic doses, there is little depression of respiration and blood pressure. Reflex systems are not depressed and the patient can be awakened easily. Generally, chloral hydrate administration is not accompanied by the "hangover effect" frequently produced by other hypnotic medications.

Chloral hydrate produces few adverse reactions other than slight gastric irritation. But because this drug easily passes the placental barrier, chloral hydrate is not recommended for pregnant women.

The hypnotic dose for adults is usually 500 mg or 1 gram, administered fifteen to thirty minutes before bedtime. Some studies have demonstrated that 500 mg of chloral hydrate is not significantly more effective than a placebo (chap. 5).

Two other derivatives, chloral betaine and triclofos sodium (fig. 2.3), possess the same hypnotic properties as chloral hydrate but do not have its unpleasant odor and taste. Unlike chloral hydrate, triclofos sodium produces many adverse reactions, including headache, hangover, drowsiness, gastrointestinal upset, nightmares, and a reduction in total white-blood-cell count. Chloral betaine, a chemical complex of chloral hydrate and betaine, has basically the same properties and actions as chloral hydrate.

Barbiturates   Although barbituric acid was first prepared in 1864 by Adolf von Bayer, its derivatives were not introduced into medicine for their hypnotic properties until 1903. Then the barbiturates quickly took over the entire world market for hypnotics and sedatives; it is likely that phenobarbital and secobarbital (under various trade names) have been used in larger quantities than any other sleeping medication in human history.

Figure 2.4 gives the basic structure of barbituric acid and a number of its derivatives. Many of them have anesthetic as well as hypnotic activities. The barbiturates are able to depress reversibly the activity of all excitable tissues studied thus far; nervous system tissues are more sensitive to the action of barbiturates than muscle tissues, but both are affected. It is believed that the barbiturates act at the synapse; they have been shown to depress the excitatory postsynaptic potential (EPSP). This may occur by action at the receptor site or by stabilization of the postsynaptic membrane, but the exact mechanisms are still unknown. In terms of neuroanatomical level, it appears that sleep is produced by barbiturates primarily through action at the level of the thalamus; here,

GENERAL FORMULA:

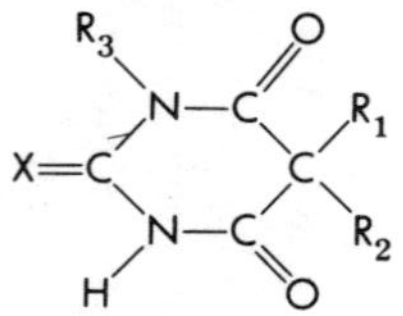

BARBITURATE	TRADE NAME	R_1	R_2	R_3	X
Amobarbital	AMYTAL	ethyl	isopentyl	H	O
Aprobarbital	ALURATE	allyl	isopropyl	H	O
Barbital	NEURONIDIA	ethyl	ethyl	H	O
Butabarbital	BUTISOL	ethyl	sec-butyl	H	O
Hexobarbital	SOMBULEX	methyl	1-cyclohexen-1-yl	CH_3	O
Mephobarbital	MEBARAL	ethyl	phenyl	CH_3	O
Metharbital	GEMONIL	ethyl	ethyl	CH_3	O
Methohexital	BREVITAL	allyl	1-methyl-2-pentynyl	CH_3	O
Pentobarbital	NEMBUTAL	ethyl	1-methylbutyl	H	O
Phenobarbital	LUMINAL	ethyl	phenyl	H	O
Probarbital	IPRAL	ethyl	isopropyl	H	O
Secobarbital	SECONAL	allyl	1-methylbutyl	H	O
Talbutal	LOTUSATE	allyl	sec-butyl	H	O
Thiamylal	SURITAL	allyl	1-methylbutyl	H	S
Thiopental	PENTOTHAL	ethyl	1-methylbutyl	H	S

Reprinted with permission from S. C. Harvey: Hypnotics and Sedatives, in Goodman, L. and Gilman, A., Eds.: *The Pharmacological Basis of Therapeutics*. New York, Macmillan 1975.

FIGURE 2.4 Barbiturates Currently Available in the U.S.A.: Names and Structures

barbiturates inhibit ascending neural impulses in the reticular formation and consequently interfere with transmission to the cortex.

The barbiturates are among the most powerful CNS depressants. In small doses they have been used as daytime sedatives, in somewhat larger doses as hypnotic agents; and in doses several times as large they act as anesthetics (in fact, they are frequently used as general anesthetics for minor operations). Doses not much higher than those used for anesthesia produce coma and eventually death. The precise effective dosage varies somewhat among the different barbiturate derivatives, but the sequence outlined above is true for all. The derivatives differ chiefly in their rapidity of onset and duration of action.

Barbiturate medication may produce a wide variety of adverse reactions, including respiratory depression, apnea, circulatory collapse, severe depression of the central nervous system, hangovers, nausea, and vomiting. Barbiturates should not ordinarily be administered to pregnant women because these drugs readily cross the placental barrier and produce a depressant effect on the fetus.

The barbiturates, though very widely used and apparently effective, have suffered from a number of serious medical problems; they have frequently been agents of abuse, suicide, and even homicide. These problems will be discussed later in connection with the risks of all hypnotic agents (chap. 8).

Paraldehyde   Paraldehyde (fig. 2.5), discovered by Vicenzo Cervello, has been used as a hypnotic since 1882. It is a colorless liquid that has a strong odor and a burning, unpleasant taste. Paraldehyde readily decomposes to acetaldehyde when exposed to light and air; subsequently this substance is oxidized to acetic acid. Administration of deteriorated paraldehyde leads to poisoning that may be fatal. Because of these various problems, paraldehyde has never achieved widespread use despite its effectiveness.

Paraldehyde is rapidly absorbed; maximum concentrations

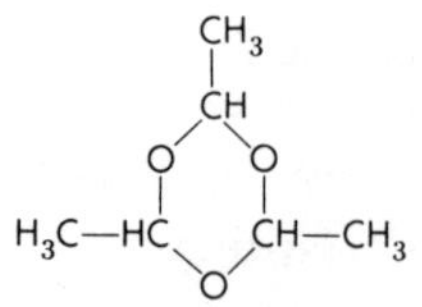

$$CH_3$$

FIGURE 2.5   Paraldehyde

in the brain are reached within thirty minutes after oral administration. Although this substance is rapidly effective in producing sleep, little is known about its pharmacological actions and metabolism.

In the usual doses, paraldehyde does not produce severe side effects. After administration of this drug, however, the patient's breath will develop a characteristic pungent odor; this is due to a small portion of paraldehyde which is excreted through the lungs. Paraldehyde ordinarily produces little respiratory depression and hypotension, but these may occur when large doses are administered. Paraldehyde can readily pass the placental barrier and depress the neural activity of the neonate.

Although this drug is seldom prescribed for ordinary insomnia, paraldehyde has found a place in the treatment of alcohol withdrawal symptoms and other abstinence syndromes. The reasons for the evolution of this specific use are not clear; it may have originated from the notion that, due to its unpleasant odor and taste, paraldehyde would be less liable to misuse.

Piperidinediones   The two best-known piperidinediones are glutethimide and methyprylon (fig. 2.6). Glutethimide,* first introduced into medicine in 1954, quickly became very popular; the dangers of the barbiturates were being

_____
* Brand name "Doriden"

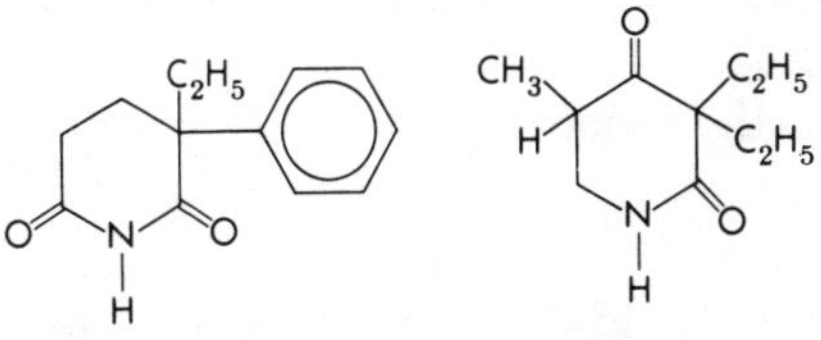

Glutethimide   Methyprylon

FIGURE 2.6   The Piperidinediones

rapidly acknowledged, and this new drug was obviously not a barbiturate. However, after a number of years, it became clear that glutethimide presented many of the same problems the barbiturates did. It is also a dangerous drug and has considerable potential for abuse. Although glutethimide is widely used, it is not certain that it has any advantages over the barbiturates.

It appears that the actions of glutethimide on various nervous system preparations are very much like the actions of the barbiturates. Although the precise mechanism of action remains unknown, it is believed that glutethimide possesses anticholinergic properties and acts primarily at the synapse.

In therapeutic doses (250 to 500 mg at bedtime) glutethimide does not produce respiratory depression. The only frequently encountered adverse reaction is a generalized skin rash which usually disappears within several days after drug withdrawal. Occasionally nausea and blurring of vision may occur.

Methyprylon* was also introduced in the 1950s and has become quite popular as another nonbarbiturate. Although it is also a piperidinedione, the pharmacological properties of methyprylon are not closely related to those of glutethimide. Very little detailed information concerning absorption, distribution, and pharmacology of methyprylon is available.

* Brand name "Nodular"

However, animal studies have shown that this piperidinedione tends to increase the threshold of arousal centers located
in the brainstem.

Although methyprylon produces few adverse reactions,
morning drowsiness, as well as gastric upset and headaches,
have been reported after the recommended dosage. The usual
adult dose for sleep induction is 200 to 400 mg at bedtime.

It is not clear that the piperidinediones offer definite advantages over the barbiturates. However, some patients, for
unknown reasons, appear to respond especially well to these
medications.

Ethchlorvynol   Ethchlorvynol* is a rapidly acting hypnotic which possesses a simple chemical structure
(fig. 2.7). In addition to its hypnotic properties, ethchlorvynol
has been used as an anticonvulsant and a muscle relaxant.

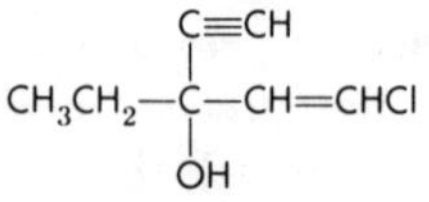

$$CH_3CH_2-\underset{\underset{OH}{|}}{\overset{\overset{C\equiv CH}{|}}{C}}-CH=CHCl$$

FIGURE 2.7   Ethchlorvynol

Absorption of ethchlorvynol from the gastrointestinal tract
is rapid; central nervous system depression occurs within fifteen to twenty minutes after oral administration, and the
maximum level in the bloodstream is obtained in approximately one and one-half hours. As with the other nonbarbiturate compounds, many of the effects of ethchlorvynol on the
nervous system are very similar to the effects of the barbiturates. More specifically, fast EEG activity initially seen in
the frontal lobes is a product of both ethchlorvynol and
barbiturate medication.

* Brand name "Placidyl"

Ethchlorvynol produces many side effects, including hypotension, nausea or vomiting, gastrointestinal upset, blurring of vision, facial numbness, and mild hangovers. Although it is not certain that there are any clear advantages in the use of ethchlorvynol, it has been accepted as a useful hypnotic by a fairly large number of physicians and patients.

Methaqualone   Methaqualone* (fig. 2.8) also has a wide range of activities: it is used as an anticonvulsant, antispasmodic and local anesthetic, and antitussor, in addition to its properties as a hypnotic.

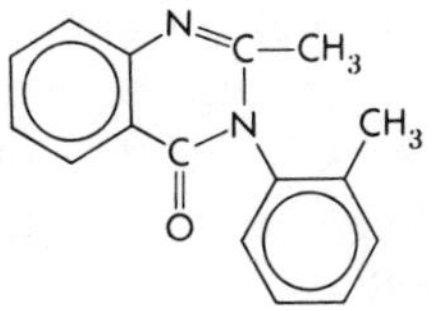

FIGURE 2.8   Methaqualone

The mechanism of action of methaqualone is not known. Overdoses produce excessive depression of the central nervous system similar to that seen with the barbiturates. Methaqualone is rapid-acting and drowsiness may occur within ten to twenty minutes after administration.

Common side effects of methaqualone include headaches, hangovers, transient paresthesia of the extremities, occasional anxiety, anorexia, nausea, and diarrhea. Currently, it is not used in women who are or may become pregnant because animal studies have revealed minor but definite skeletal abnormalities in the offspring. Methaqualone is toxic in high doses; acute overdosage may cause delirium, coma, and convulsions. It has recently become a drug of widespread abuse.

* Brand name "Quaalude," "Sopor"

The Benzodiazepines   This class of drugs is now among the most frequently prescribed of all drugs in the United States. The benzodiazepines include chlordiazepoxide,* diazepam,† flurazepam,‡ nitrazepam,§ and a number of other similar agents soon to be introduced into medical practice. They are used as antianxiety agents and as hypnotics. The benzodiazepines as a group have a number of interesting effects on the central nervous system. The exact mode of action has not been specified; they presumably act at central nervous system synapses, and it has been suggested that they may specifically affect either gamma-amino butyric acid (GABA) or glycine synapses. In some animal studies, flurazepam reduced responses to electrical stimulation of the hypothalamus and increased the arousal threshold of both the amgydala and the hypothalamus. Although in many ways the benzodiazepines are central nervous system depressants, their activity does differ in some ways from that of the barbiturates and other depressants; therefore, they are often referred to as "tranquilizers" rather than sedatives or hypnotics.

Flurazepam hydrochloride (fig. 2.9) is most frequently prescribed as a hypnotic. However, since the actions of the

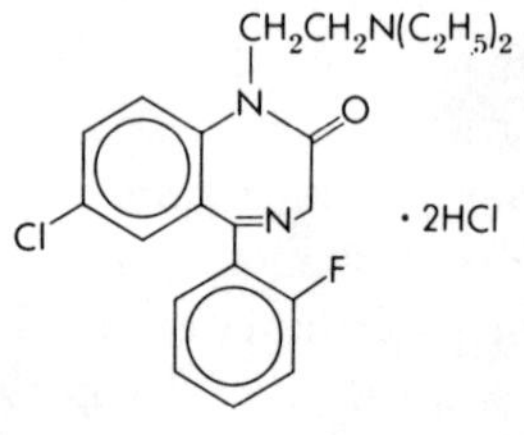

FIGURE 2.9   Flurazepam Hydrochloride

* Brand name "Librium"
† Brand name "Valium"
‡ Brand name "Dalmane"
§ Brand name "Mogadon"

other benzodiazepines are extremely similar, they can in fact all be used as hypnotic agents. The benzodiazepines have some of the same problems encountered with other hypnotics: they produce many adverse side effects, including headaches, heartburn, gastroirritation, palpitations, chest pains, body and joint pains. In addition, sweating, difficulty in focusing, blurred vision, burning eyes, hypotension, shortness of breath, skin rash, dry mouth, anorexia, depression, confusion, and hallucinations have been reported. Also, the benzodiazepines have disturbing interactions with other depressants—including alcohol.

However, the benzodiazepines possess one great advantage over the barbiturates and the nonbarbiturates discussed thus far: the therapeutic index is extremely high. In other words, it is almost impossible to die from an overdose of benzodiazepines. Apparently they do not produce increasing central nervous system depression with increasing dosage; and they produce little or no respiratory depression.

Antihistamines   Although the antihistamines are not usually listed in textbooks as hypnotic agents, they clearly possess sleep-inducing properties. In fact, two antihistamines, diphenhydramine and methapyrilene (fig. 2.10), are widely used as hypnotics. Methapyrilene is possibly the most widely used hypnotic agent in the United States (chap. 3) but the

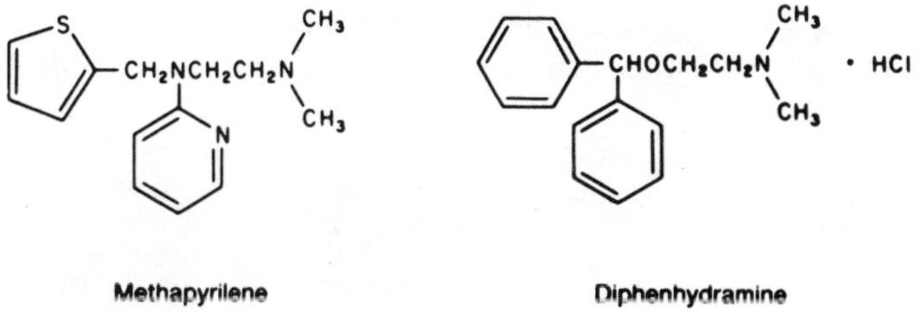

Methapyrilene   Diphenhydramine

FIGURE 2.10 *Two Antihistamines: Methapyrilene; Diphenhydramine*

reasons are somewhat accidental: the laws regulating over-the-counter (nonprescription) medication are such that methapyrilene was included under a "grandfather clause," whereas most other antihistamines, including some more effective ones, were not included; thus, nearly all available over-the-counter hypnotic agents depend on the activity of methapyrilene.*

Although methapyrilene is widely used, it is not the antihistamine with the greatest hypnotic effect. Diphenhydramine is an ethanolamine and probably the antihistamine with the clearest hypnotic effects. However, diphenhydramine is not an especially powerful hypnotic; it is relatively safe and free of side effects, and is consequently often used in cases where a mild drug is needed, for instance, for children and the aged. The mechanism of the hypnotic action is uncertain; it appears not to be related to the histamine-blocking effects of the antihistamines.

Although methapyrilene and diphenhydramine are both relatively safe drugs their widespread availability has made accidental poisoning by overdose fairly common. The predominant symptom in poisoning is excitation, including hallucinations, incoordination, and sometimes convulsions.

CONCLUSIONS

The list of hypnotic agents I have presented here is not entirely complete; a number of lesser-known agents have already been introduced into medicine, and new agents are being introduced frequently.

Overall, a strikingly heterogeneous group of compounds is

---

* In fact, I recently served for several years on a panel of the Food and Drug Administration which considered all these medications. We specifically recommended that scopolamine and the analgesics be removed from "night-time sleeping aids" (hypnotics). However, since methapyrilene appeared to have mild hypnotic effects, we suggested that, as a single ingredient, it be kept as a possible over-the-counter hypnotic. In addition, we suggested that diphenhydramine might be used over the counter, since it is just as safe and probably more effective.

being used to improve sleep. Their chemical structures makes it clear that these substances are very different from one another; it is quite likely that they act on a number of very different receptors, at different sites of action, and produce a common result through quite disparate mechanisms. Furthermore, the common result, as I shall discuss later, is not specifically sleep, but rather central nervous system depression.

References

Adams, Francis, ed. and transl. *The Extant Works of Aretaeus, the Cappadocian.* London: The Sydenham Society, 1856.

American Medical Association Department of Drugs. *AMA Drug Evaluations.* 3d ed. Littleton, Mass.: Publishing Sciences Group, 1977.

Celsus. *De medicina,* with an English translation by W. G. Spencer. Vol. 1. London: William Heinemann, 1935.

Domino, E. F. Sites of action of some central nervous depressants. *Ann. Rev. Pharmacol.* 2 (1962): 215–50.

Garattini, S.; E. Mussini; and L. O. Randall, eds. *The Benzodiazepines.* New York: Raven Press, 1973.

Goldstein, A.; L. Aronow; and S. M. Kalman. *Principles of Drug Action: The Basis of Pharmacology.* 2d ed. New York: Wiley, 1974.

Goodman, Louis S., and Alfred Gilman, eds. *The Pharmacological Basis of Therapeutics.* 5th ed. New York: Macmillan, 1975.

Robinson, Victor. *Victory Over Pain.* New York: Henry Schuman, 1946.

Theophrastus. *Enquiry Into Plants,* with an English translation by Sir Arthur Hoyt. London: William Heinemann, 1916.

Wesson, Donald R., and David E. Smith. *Barbiturates: Their Use, Misuse and Abuse.* New York: Human Sciences Press, 1977.

3

Who Uses How Much of What?

There is absolutely no question that a great many sleeping pills are consumed every year, though the lack of any single, standard reporting source makes it difficult to estimate the total exactly. From various sources, one can derive figures in the following range: 10–30 percent of the population reports some difficulty in sleeping during the course of the year. Over half of these people take a sleeping pill at some time during the year. Meaningful estimates of overall use are not easy to compile, since hypnotic medication is obtained by the consumer (patient) from at least three different legal sources, as well as some illegal ones.

First, most hospital in patients take sleeping pills at some time during their hospitalization. Close to half of all hospital admissions for adults include a prescription for a sleeping pill: the medication is usually ordered *prn* (*pro re nata*), meaning that the patient can ask for and receive a particular sleeping pill at night whenever he needs it. This practice accounts for several million prescriptions per year.

Second, sleeping-pill prescriptions are written by physicians in private practice or in clinics and filled by U.S. pharmacies and drugstores. Here fairly accurate figures are available through the National Prescription Audit. There was a gradual increase in the annual number of prescriptions for hypnotic medication through 1970; from 1970 to 1973 a plateau was reached at a total of about 38 million prescriptions during the course of a year (table 3.1). Since the average prescription was written for thirty doses, this source alone accounts for over one billion doses of sleeping medications per year.

The third major route involves the direct purchase of OTC

TABLE 3.1

Hypnotics: Number of Prescriptions Filled in U.S. Drugstores, 1964–1973

		DRUG CATEGORY *			
		Hypnotics			
	Hyp-notics	Barbitu-rates	Nonbar-biturates	All psy-chotropes	All drugs
1964	29.4	(15.9)	(13.6)	149.2	857.5
1965	31.8	(17.2)	(18.0)	161.0	966.8
1966	35.7	(17.8)	(14.6)	173.9	1,054.9
1967	33.4	(17.2)	(16.2)	173.6	1,068.7
1968	33.8	(17.4)	(16.4)	185.1	1,145.4
1969	35.9	(18.2)	(17.7)	202.1	1,196.9
1970	37.5	(17.9)	(19.6)	214.4	1,279.9
1971	39.6	(17.4)	(22.3)	217.8	1,351.4
1972	38.7	(15.7)	(23.0)	214.5	1,450.5
1973	37.5	(13.8)	(23.7)	223.3	1,532.0
Change 1964–1973 (percent)	28	−13	74	50	79

* New and refill prescriptions (numbers in millions)

Source: National Prescription Audit, IMS America, Ltd.

(over-the-counter) sleeping pills by the patient or consumer. According to the National Survey on Drug Acquisition and Use, in 1970–71 6 percent of the adult population used OTC sleeping pills during the course of the year, whereas 3.5 percent used drugstore prescription hypnotics. It has been found that there is very little overlap between OTC users and drugstore prescription users: a person uses one source or the other but seldom both. This implies that close to 9.5 percent of the population uses sleeping pills from these two sources; adding those who use sleeping pills only in a hospital, it is likely that at least 10 percent of the entire adult population uses sleeping pills at some time during the year.

In addition to these legal methods of acquiring sleeping pills, a large number of pills are either stolen, imported, obtained illegally from manufacturers, or synthesized for "street use." It is very difficult to estimate the extent of this use, but some sources have suggested that several million persons have at least one experience with a sleeping pill ("downer") in the course of a year.

Since I could find no published figures for overall totals, I have made a rough attempt to estimate the total doses of sleeping pills consumed per year from all these sources combined. Both by adding up known sources of consumption of drugs (above), and alternatively, by multiplying the market in dollars by an estimate of the average cost of a pill to the consumer, I have arrived at a conservative estimate of at least three billion doses of sleeping medication used in the United States per year.

Actually, the total use of these drugs is even greater than this. We have so far considered their use only as hypnotics or sedatives—that is, to induce or improve sleep or to produce sedation and drowsiness. However, some of the same compounds have other, more specfic uses: for instance, large quantities of barbiturates, especially phenobarbital, are used in the treatment of epilepsy, and several barbiturates are used as anesthetic agents. Also, many persons taking drugs such as diazepam (Valium) use them as sleeping pills, but these have not been included in my estimate since the prescription is for a "tranquilizer."

The next question to consider is how much of what hypnotic medication is taken; these figures are available, but the figures change greatly from year to year. For 1973, relatively complete figures show that, of prescriptions filled in U.S. drugstores, 37 percent were for barbiturates and 63 percent for nonbarbiturates. (The most common nonbarbiturates were flurazepam, glutethimide, methaqualone, chloral hydrate, ethchlorvynol, and methyprylon; see table 3.2.) Since 1973 there appears to have been some further reduction in the use of barbiturates. In the over-the-counter market the most common drug by far is the antihistamine methapyrilene, usually in combination with an analgesic and sometimes in combination with other agents as well.

TABLE 3.2

Hypnotics: Number of Prescriptions for Selected Drugs Filled in U.S. Drugstores, 1964–1973

Drug subclass and drug	New and refill prescriptions (numbers in millions)									
	1964	1965	1966	1967	1968	1969	1970	1971	1972	1973
Barbiturates										
Pentobarbital	5.9	6.7	6.9	5.9	6.6	7.1	6.9	6.4	6.1	5.2
Secobarbital	6.8	6.3	6.9	7.1	6.8	6.9	6.9	6.6	5.6	5.0
Amobarbital & secobarbital	3.2	4.1	3.9	4.2	4.0	4.1	4.1	3.8	3.6	3.1
Nonbarbiturates										
Chloral hydrate	2.5	2.8	3.1	2.9	2.7	3.3	3.7	3.9	3.5	3.3
Flurazepam	—	—	—	—	—	—	0.7	2.9	4.5	6.5
Glutethimide	6.7	6.6	7.8	6.0	6.2	6.2	6.0	5.6	4.5	4.2
Methyprylon	1.2	1.4	2.2	2.4	2.6	3.0	2.8	2.5	2.4	2.2
Methaqualone	—	—	0.1	0.3	0.6	1.3	2.5	3.4	4.7	4.0
Ethchlorvynol	2.4	2.9	3.2	3.5	3.4	3.4	3.4	3.2	2.9	2.8

Source: National Prescription Audit, IMS America, Ltd.

We can ask more specific questions as to who uses these medications and who supplies them. For the answers, I have relied heavily upon the National Survey on Drug Acquisition and Use and an excellent article by Balter and Bauer (see References to this chapter). Table 3.3 estimates the total

TABLE 3.3

Use of Sleep Medication during the Year by Age, Drug Category, and Sex, 1970-1971

Drug category and sex	Age (% of age group)				
	18–29	30–34	45–59	60–74	All ages
Prescription hypnotics					
Male	1	1	2	7	3
Female	3	3	4	8	4
OTC sleeping pills					
Male	8	4	3	7	6
Female	7	7	4	5	6

Source: National Survey on Drug Acquisition and Use, 1970–71.

hypnotic drug use by age and sex. It is obvious that legal use of hypnotic medication goes up with increase in age, and that women use hypnotic medication somewhat more than do men. Table 3.4 makes it clear that prescription medications are used far more regularly than OTC medications; the latter, as expected, are used sporadically.

For drugs obtained by prescription at drugstores, information about prescribers is also available. Table 3.5 lists the specialties of the doctors prescribing sleeping medications and whether they prescribe primarily barbiturate or nonbarbiturate sleeping pills. Not surprisingly, it turns out that general practitioners and internists together write 60 percent of all sleeping-pill prescriptions. The ratio of barbiturate to nonbarbiturate prescriptions is higher for general practitioners than for internists, indicating that the latter group, by 1973, may have become more concerned about problems with barbiturates and more likely to change to newer substitutes.

TABLE 3.4

Comparison of Users of Prescription Hypnotics with Users of Over-the-Counter Sleeping Pills on Level of Use, 1970–1971

Level of use	Prescription hypnotics users (% distribution)*	Over-the-counter sleeping pill users (% distribution)*
High (daily use, 2 months or more)	23	2
Medium (daily use, 1 week–2 months or 31 occasions)	33	15
Low (daily use, less than 1 week or fewer than 31 occasions)	44	81
Total	100	100
Number of persons	(104)	(142)

* Columns may not add to 100% because of rounding.

Source: National Survey on Drug Acquisition and Use, 1970–71.

The prescription of hypnotics is relatively concentrated: the 10 percent of physicians who write the most prescriptions accounts for 35 percent of the yearly total sleeping-pill prescriptions. Balter and Bauer suggest that the number of prescriptions for hypnotics tends to be strongly correlated with the size of the physician's practice: physicians who see the largest number of patients tend to prescribe the most hypnotics; it is likely but not certain from the data that they prescribe more hypnotics *per patient seen.*

Statistical information is sketchy on the question of diagnostic category—just why sleeping pills are prescribed. They are clearly prescribed for many medical and surgical conditions associated with sleep disorders: these accounted for 50 percent of sleeping-pill prescriptions (table 3.6). However, the other half of the prescriptions were for "sleep disturbance," "mental disorders," or "special conditions without sickness." The diagnostic category "symptoms and senility" in

TABLE 3.5

Distribution of Hypnotic Drug Prescribing by
Specialty of Physician, 1973

Specialty	Physicians in private practice°	Hypnotics (% distribution)		
		Total	Barbitu-rates	Nonbar-biturates
General practitioner	31	39	40	39
Internist	16	21	11	25
Surgeon	16	10	12	9
Obstetrician/gynecologist	8	10	13	9
Psychiatrist/neurologist	6	7	5	8
Pediatrician	6	4	9	3
Osteopath	7	5	6	5
All others	10	3	6	3
Total	100	100	100	100

° Columns may not add to 100% because of rounding.

Source: National Disease and Therapeutic Index, IMS America, Ltd.,
      1973.

Table 3.6 is a catch-all used by The National Disease and
Therapeutic Index that does not seem especially useful. As is
evident from the table, most prescriptions in this category
were apparently for "sleep disturbance" with no more specific
diagnosis given. I shall discuss the classification and etiology
of sleep disturbance in detail in chapter 8.

The very thorough survey by Balter and Bauer (1975)
concludes that, overall, the picture is "an essentially conservative" one of responsible behavior: they feel that "a
rather small proportion of the population uses hypnotic drugs
during the course of the year [10%] and usually for only a
short period of time." Also, Balter and Bauer find that use has
not increased significantly between 1964 and 1973, or at least
that the use of hypnotic medication has not increased faster
than the total increase in visits to physicians.

I would agree that probably most of the use of hypnotic
medication by doctors and patients can be considered "responsible." However, this does not indicate to me that all is
well. Ten percent of the population comprises a very large

TABLE 3.6

New Therapy: Distribution of Hypnotic Drug Prescribing by
Diagnostic Category and Drug Subclass, 1973

Diagnostic Category	Barbiturate hypnotic (% distribution)°	Nonbarbiturate hypnotic (% distribution)°	Total hypnotics (% distribution)°
"Symptoms and senility"	19	24	22
Sleep disturbance	(12)	(19)	(17)
Convulsive and neurological	(4)	(—)	(1)
Other	(3)	(5)	(4)
Mental disorders	15	22	20
Special conditions without sickness	13	9	10
Circulatory disorders	6	10	9
Disorders of respiratory system	10	8	8
Disorders of bones and organs of movement	2	5	4
Delivery and complications of pregnancy	4	4	4
Digestive disorders	4	3	3
Genitourinary disorders	2	3	3
Neoplasms	6	3	3
Disorders of the CNS sense organs	8	2	4
Accident and poisoning	8	2	4
Disorders of skin and cellular tissue	1	2	2
Allergic, metabolic, nutritional disorders	1	2	2
Blood and blood-forming organs	—	1	1
Infective and parasitic diseases	2	—	1
Total	100	100	100

° Columns may not add to 100% because of rounding.

Source: National Disease and Therapeutic Index, IMS America, Ltd.,
1973.

number of people. Even a small percentage, say 10–30 percent, of irresponsible use represents a huge number of dangerous situations. And "responsible" use apparently means
only that prescriptions for hypnotics have not risen out of
sight in recent years. "Responsibility" on the part of the

doctor by no means indicates that the sleeping pills prescribed are anything close to ideal medications. In fact, as we shall see, they produce numerous dangers or problems. And a statistical overview can give us little indication of how many of the millions who took prescription or nonprescription sleeping pills might have been better off with some other form of treatment.

Finally, I believe that the concentration of sleeping-pill prescriptions mentioned above, and the especially high number of prescriptions by the busiest physicians, are worth commenting on. The fact that the physician who sees more patients prescribes more hypnotics is in itself hardly surprising. Obviously a physician who sees more patients will, on the average, see more patients with sleep problems and thus, on the average, may prescribe more sleeping pills. However, I do not believe this is the whole story. Though it is difficult to prove absolutely, I am quite certain from the above figures and from my own observations, that patients with sleep problems are far more likely to have a sleeping pill prescribed if their physician has only ten minutes to spend with them than if he has thirty or forty minutes, or more. Ten minutes is just not time enough to explore the causes of insomnia and the various possible treatments of its underlying causes.

References

Balter, M. B., and M. L. Bauer. Patterns of prescribing and use of hypnotic drugs in the United States. In *Sleep Disturbance and Hypnotic Drug Dependence*, edited by A. D. Clift, pp. 261–93. Amsterdam: Excerpta Medica, 1975.

Karacan, I.; J. I. Thornby; M. Anch; et al. Prevalence of sleep disturbance in a primarily urban Florida county, *Social Science Medicine* 10 (1976): 239–44.

Mellinger, G. D.; M. B. Balter; H. J. Parry; D. I. Manheimer; and I. H. Cisin. In E. Josephson and E. E. Carroll, eds., *Drug Use— Epidemiological and Sociological Approaches*, chap. 15, pp. 333–36. Washington, D.C.: Hemisphere Publishing Corporation, 1974.

National Center for Health Statistics Current Estimates from the *Health Interview Survey, United States,* ser. 10, no. 94. Washington, D.C.: U.S. Government Printing Office, 1973.

National Prescription Audit, IMS America, 1973.

Parry, H. J.; M. B. Balter; et al. National patterns of psychotherapeutic drug use. *Archives of General Psychiatry* 28 (1973): 769–83.

4

Sleep

In the following chapters we shall consider important questions to which we can give lengthy but not entirely complete answers. The primary questions are: Do sleeping pills work—do they actually put people to sleep? Is the state they induce actual sleep or is it something very different? In other words, what effects do sleeping pills actually have on sleep? Also, what other effects do they have on people who take them in addition to "putting them to sleep"? Do the beneficial effects of sleeping pills outweigh the risks?

In order to answer these questions I shall first discuss some basic aspects of sleep, including sleep physiology, sleep chemistry, sleep pathology, and the possible functions of sleep. I shall then consider laboratory and clinical studies that have investigated the effects of sleeping pills (chap. 5) and go on to discuss insomnia and its treatment in later chapters.

SLEEP DEFINED

Although the term *sleep research* now appropriately summons up visions of complex polygraphic apparatus, sleep is basically a behavioral state. It is a regular, recurrent, easily reversible state of the organism characterized by relative quiescence and a great increase in threshold of response to external stimuli (relative to the waking state). Thus the definition of sleep is behavioral.

However, certain EEG and polygraphic characteristics can now be accepted as part of a definition of sleep because of their regular and constant association with the behavior called sleep. Yet it is worth emphasizing that the changes often considered characteristic of sleep may be deceptive. For instance, the deep slow waves usually associated with sleep can be found in the waking state under certain pharmacological conditions and also during certain phases of anesthesia or coma. Thus, when the EEG tracing is used to make the "diagnosis" of sleep, it is the regular patterning rather than any single characteristic wave-form which is most important.

METHODS OF STUDYING SLEEP

There has been interest for a great many years in studying the amount, depth, "quality," and so on, of sleep from the clinical point of view in following the course of a mental or physical illness, as well as in evaluating sleeping medications. A variety of techniques has been employed. One classic method is simply the subjective report: the doctor, for instance, simply asks the patient whether he or she has been sleeping better or worse than usual. This simple and inexpensive way of evaluating sleep is widely used and not to be denigrated; it can be refined to a certain extent by the use of questionnaires that ask specific questions of interest. Although the information obtained from subjective reports is sensitive to many sources of bias, it nonetheless supplies information not obtainable by any other means: quite obviously a sleeping medication, let us say, which looked perfect from the point of view of various objective studies but left the patient feeling miserable in the morning would be a poor medication indeed.

One method used to supplement the sometimes biased subjective reports involves the use of an objective observer who checks the patient or subject at stated intervals—say every fifteen or thirty minutes during the night—and categorizes his observations, for example, as: Awake, Asleep, Not certain. This method has the advantage that it can be applied to a large number of sleeping persons at the same time, at relatively low expense; and such observations have been found to correlate fairly closely with EEG measures of sleep, except in certain problematic cases such as the sleep of depressed patients in the early morning hours.

During the 1930s and 1940s a popular technique for measuring length and depth of sleep was to attach a simple movement-sensitive device to the subject's bedsprings, and simply to record the amount of bed motion during the night. This is based on the somewhat oversimplified notion that sleep can be gauged simply by diminution of movement and that the deepest sleep is the sleep involving the least motion. Still, these studies did lead to at least rough estimates of changes in the length of sleep and to a general notion that the early hours of sleep are the deepest, at least in the sense of containing the least movement. These observations, as far as they go, are still valid.

More recently, EEG and polygraphic studies of sleep have become the dominant method of study. These involve continuous measurement of relevant variables—most commonly the occipital and parietal electroencephalogram (EEG), eye movements, muscle potential, and in certain cases the electrocardiogram (EKG), measures of respiration, etc. This method has the obvious advantage of providing a continuous minute-by-minute record of the entire night's sleep. Among the disadvantages of this technique are expense and the fact that application of the necessary electrodes for recording may be somewhat disturbing to sleep, requiring one, two, or in certain cases more nights of "adaptation" to the sleep laboratory before an accurate evaluation of sleep can be made.

A TYPICAL NIGHT'S SLEEP

The following description provides a brief summary of the phenomenology of sleep—what occurs during a typical night of sleep in a young adult. A great deal of the information here is derived from recent polygraphic studies, but many of the findings are amenable to study by the various other techniques described, including visual observation.

As the subject in the sleep laboratory falls asleep, his brain waves go through certain characteristic changes, usually classified as stages 1, 2, 3, and 4. Waking EEG is characterized by alpha waves (8–12 cycles per second) and low-voltage activity of mixed frequency. As the subject falls asleep, she or he begins to show a disappearance of alpha activity. Stage 1, considered the lightest stage of sleep, is characterized by low-voltage desynchronized activity and sometimes by low-voltage, regular 4–6 cycle-per-second activity as well. After a few seconds or minutes this gives way to stage 2, a pattern showing chiefly frequent 13–15 cycle-per-second spindle-shaped tracings, known as sleep spindles, and by certain high-voltage spikes known as K-complexes. In a few more minutes delta waves, high-voltage activity at 0.5–2 cycles per second, make their appearance (stage 3), and eventually these delta waves occupy the major part of the record (fig. 4.1).

Sleep is cyclical, with four or five periods of "emergence" from stages 2, 3, and 4 to a stage similar to stage 1 (fig. 4.2). These periods during the night are associated with frequent dream recall and are characterized not only by stage 1 EEG and by rapid conjugate eye movements, but by a host of other factors which distinguish them from the remainder of sleep. Among these factors are a great irregularity in pulse rate, respiratory rate, and blood pressure; the presence of full or partial penile erections in the male; and a general muscular atony interrupted only by sporadic movements in small muscle groups. These four or five periods during the night are not typical stage 1 as found at sleep onset; in fact, they are so different from the remainder of sleep, in the ways described above and also in terms of their neurophysiology and chemistry, that they are now almost universally considered a separate "state" of sleep. This view is reinforced by the fact that similar periods differing markedly from the remainder of sleep are found in all, or almost all, mammals and birds studied. We refer to these periods of desynchronized sleep as *D* (for desynchronized or dreaming) *sleep* and the remainder of sleep as *S* (synchronized) *sleep*. These same two states are

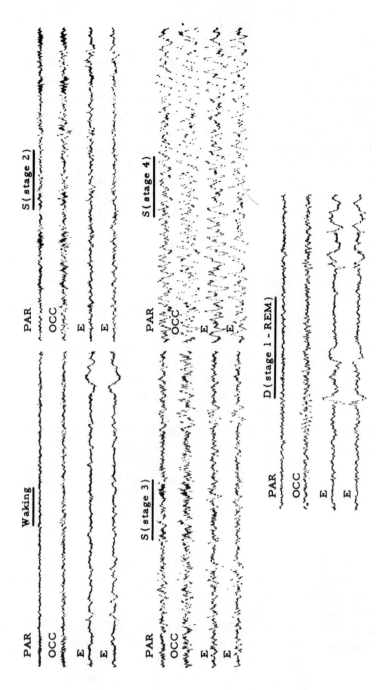

FIGURE 4.1 EEG and Eye-Movement Records

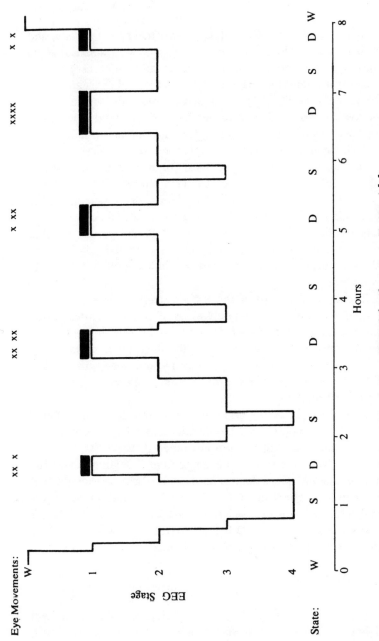

FIGURE 4.2 A Typical Night's Sleep in a Young Adult

also referred to as *REM* (rapid eye movement) *sleep* and *NREM* (nonrapid eye movement) *sleep*; as *paradoxical sleep* and *orthodox sleep*; or as *active sleep* and *quiet sleep*.

Several important characteristics of the night's sleep should be noted (see fig. 4.2). First of all, there are typically four or five D-periods during the night, and the total time taken up by these periods, or D-time, is about one and a half hours, a little over 20 percent of total sleep time. There is some variation, of course, but the most interesting fact is that all of the thousands of human subjects studied have such D-periods and these almost always take up 20–25 percent of the total night's sleep. The first D-period occurs about ninety to one hundred minutes after the onset of sleep; this interval may be longer in some normal subjects, but it is significantly shorter only under a few unusual clinical and experimental conditions.

The cyclical nature of the night's sleep is quite regular: a D-period occurs approximately every 90 to 100 minutes during the night. The first D-period tends to be the shortest, often lasting only five or six minutes, while the later D-periods may last twenty to forty minutes. Most D-time occurs in the last third of the night, whereas most stage 4 sleep occurs in the first third of the night.

S-sleep can be neatly organized according to depth. Stage 1 is the lightest and stage 4 the deepest stage, by arousal threshold measures as well as by appearance of the EEG. D-sleep, however, does not fit into this continuum. Looking only at the human electroencephalographic data, it might be thought that D-sleep is a light sleep. Yet the arousal threshold in animals is higher in D- than in S-sleep, and resting muscle potential is lowest during D. Thus, D is neither truly light sleep nor deep sleep but a qualitatively *different* kind of sleep.

The Phylogeny of Sleep

According to our behavioral definition of sleep, most vertebrates—certainly reptiles, birds, and mammals—may be said to display some form of sleep.

Reptiles show behavioral sleep and have slow frequencies in the cortex resembling mammalian S-sleep; in a few instances, brief episodes of a state very much resembling D-sleep have been recorded as well. Birds have definite periods of both S- and D-sleep, although the D-periods are short and account for a very small percentage of total sleep time.

Within the class Mammalia the two states of sleep have been studied in a wide variety of different species. Probably all or almost all mammals have S- and D-sleep. However, it has been reported that D-sleep is absent in a single very primitive mammal, the spiny anteater. If indeed this mammal is found not to experience D-sleep, this could have important implications as to when the differentiation of the two states of sleep arose phylogenetically. Also, it is interesting that this mammal has a surprisingly complicated-looking brain (very convoluted cerebral brain hemispheres) for an otherwise primitive species. It has been suggested that D-sleep might be an innovation allowing later mammals to perform more efficiently whatever tasks the anteater's elaborate hemispheres perform.

No very obvious relationships among species are evident in terms of amounts of S- or D-sleep. The so-called higher mammals, such as man and apes, do not show either more or less sleep or more or less D-time than the "lower" forms. Within closely related species, for instance among the rodents, animals which are usually preyed upon (for example, rabbits) have less D-time than the predators (rats). To some extent this is true across many groups of mammals: carnivores tend to have more D-time than herbivores with the omnivores in between. This makes sense from the point of view of adaptation and selection, since the muscular relaxation of the D-state would make an animal especially vulnerable during this time, and long D-periods would be especially disadvantageous to herbivores and to preyed upon animals.

There is a definite relationship between the basal metabolic rate of a species and the length of the sleep-dream cycle (usually defined as the time from the end of one D-period to the end of the next). Smaller mammals with higher metabolic rates, such as the mouse, have shorter sleep-dream cycles; there is an inverse relationship between the metabolic rate of the species and the sleep-dream-cycle length (fig. 4.3). Indeed, the same relationship can be found between metabolic rate and the length of the pulse cycle, the respiratory cycle, the gestation period, and the life span. These data help to establish the fact that the sleep-dream cycle is one of the basic cycles of the mammalian body.

THE ONTOGENY OF THE
SLEEP STATES

One of the most consistent findings of recent sleep studies is that the young always have more sleep time, and considerably more D-time, than the adults of the species. The young adult human spends sixteen to seventeen hours awake and seven to eight hours asleep; of the seven to eight hours of sleep, perhaps six hours of sleep time are spent in S-sleep and one and a half hours in D-sleep. Both S and D are, on the average, slightly reduced with increasing age. The newborn child spends sixteen to eighteen hours asleep, and at least half of his sleep is spent in the D-state. Although exact definition and scoring of S and D are somewhat problematic in very young children, this finding has been made repeatedly and suggests that D-sleep is an especially primitive state. The same ontogenetic relationship appears to hold for other mammalian species. The young mammal always sleeps more than the adult and has an especially high percentage of D-time. Also, the sleep-dream cycle is clearly present at birth and is generally shorter in the newborn child or animal than in the adult of the same species.

THE NEUROPHYSIOLOGY
OF SLEEP

It is impossible to do justice here to this complex and very important area. Several references listed (see pp. 57–59) will help the interested reader.

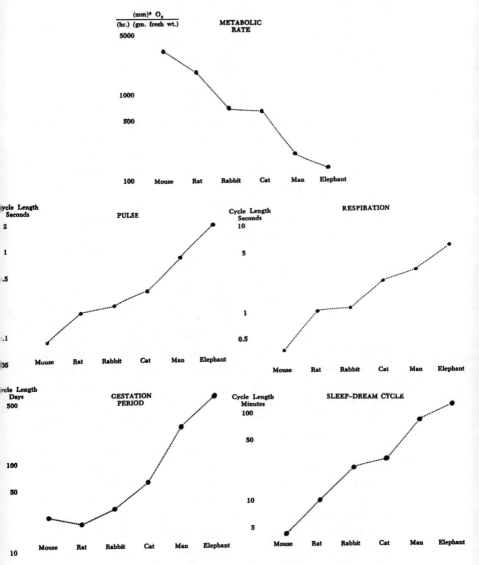

FIGURE 4.3   Basal Metabolic Rate and Length of Cycles
in Six Mammalian Species

Maintenance of the waking state depends on the activity of the ascending reticular activating system (ARAS), which sends impulses to the forebrain. For some time after discovery of the ARAS, it was assumed that sleep supervened simply when ARAS activity fell below a certain level ("passive theory" of sleep). It now appears that there are several active processes subserving sleep. Synchronized sleep in animals probably depends on activity of certain centers in the brainstem, especially the raphe nuclei, as well as certain areas in the medial forebrain; and other areas in the hypothalamus and the thalamus cannot be entirely excluded. The important serotonin-containing raphe system will be discussed again later. It is possible that at sleep onset these sleep-inducing systems exert an influence on ARAS activity or compete with it for effect on the rest of the brain.

In addition, there is a brainstem system necessary for the initiating and maintenance of D-sleep. This involves parts of the pontine brainstem: Portions of the *locus coerulus* contribute to the muscular inhibition characteristic of D-sleep. Neurons in the giganto-cellular tegmental fields (FTG) of the brainstem tegmentum also may play a prominent role: they greatly increase their firing rates at the beginning or just before the beginning of a D-period; thus, this area may be considered an *initiator* or *pacemaker* for D-sleep. It has been suggested by Hobson and McCarley (1975) that the FTG and *locus coerulus* may control the states of sleep by a process of reciprocal inhibition.

In any case, there is no question that the two states of sleep are distinct states neurophysiologically. In the many species studied, S-sleep is characterized overall by relatively "inactivated" patterns in most parts of the brain; recordings from single neurons in most areas demonstrate lower firing rates than during waking. During D-sleep most areas show "activated" patterns, and single neurons have a firing rate as high or higher than during active wakefulness.

NEUROCHEMISTRY OF SLEEP

The total chemistry of mammalian sleep is also a complex subject, but it is worth discussing in some detail here, since one would expect that the chemistry of sleeping pills ought to bear some relationship to that of sleep. As we shall see, this has so far not been the case.

There are at least three different chemical systems or groups of systems that have been shown to be definitely related to sleep. Perhaps the most important system involves brain serotonin, which is contained almost entirely in neurons with their cell bodies in the raphe nuclei of the brainstem, and with axons terminating in widespread areas of the brain—the brainstem as well as higher brain centers (fig. 4.4). In cats, almost total sleeplessness can be produced either by lesions of the raphe nuclei (which drastically reduce brain serotonin), or by interference with the synthesis of serotonin by administering PCPA, a blocker of tryptophan hydroxylase, which prevents the synthesis of serotonin from tryptophan. When brain serotonin levels remain at a low level, sleep begins to return, but it is a rather abnormal sleep. My laboratory has demonstrated that administration of l-tryptophan, which is perhaps the most physiological way of increasing levels of brain serotonin where it normally occurs in the brain, definitely induces sleep in animals and in man (see chapter 10).

In addition, brain catecholamines are important to the maintenance of wakefulness. The catecholamines are a group of organic compounds with a phenol nucleus, including two hydroxyl groups on the phenol ring. My discussion will be limited to two important brain catecholamines, dopamine and norepinephrine (fig. 4.5). It has long been recognized that the ARAS is involved in the maintenance of wakefulness and alertness. It turns out that much of this effect may be due to more specifically delineated pathways within the ARAS containing cells which release dopamine or norepinephrine at their endings. Many pharmacological studies indicate that the catecholamines play a definite role in producing arousal.

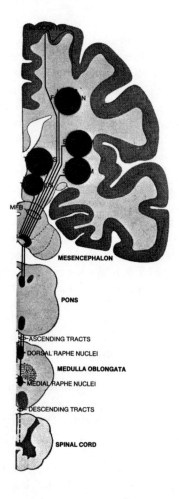

Diagrammatic representation of serotonergic (5-HT)
pathways arising in the mesencephalon, entering the median
forebrain bundle (mfb) and innervating rostral nuclei.

FIGURE 4.4 Brain Serotonin Pathways

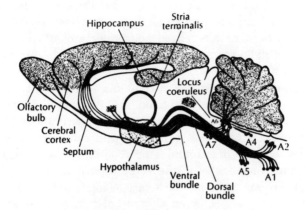

Brain Norepinephrine Pathways

Sagittal projection of the ascending NE pathways. The
descending pathways are not included. The shaded areas
indicate the major nerve terminal areas.

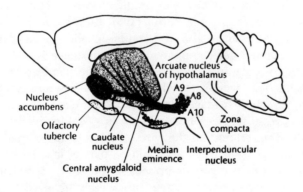

Brain Dopamine Pathways

Sagittal projection of the DA pathways. The shaded
areas indicate nerve terminal areas.

FIGURE 4.5 Brain Norepinephrine Pathways; Brain
Dopamine Pathways

I have argued at length elsewhere that there is an important difference between the two amines: dopamine appears to be involved in more generalized nonspecific arousal or pressure, while ascending norepinephrine systems may be involved in aspects such as focused attention during waking.

Thus sleep, compared to wakefulness, would involve both an increase in functional serotonin activity and a decrease in functional dopamine and/or norepinephrine. Radulovacki and his coworkers have shown that sleep in cats is characterized by an increase in serotonin metabolites and a decrease in dopamine metabolites in the cerebrospinal fluid. I shall discuss later some ways in which various forms of insomnia could result from changes, or an altered balance, in these systems.

A third aspect of the chemistry of sleep has been much studied but is difficult to relate to the above neurochemistry. A group led by Monnier in Switzerland (1964, 1974) has found a substance—a short-chain peptide—in the blood of sleep-deprived animals, which can produce sleep in other animals. Pappenheimer's group in Boston (1967, 1975) has found a sleep-inducing substance—also a peptide—in the spinal fluid of sleep-deprived goats. Apparently the substance is not found, or occurs only in minute quantities, in nonsleep-deprived animals. This work is solid: such substances apparently do exist, though their exact role in sleep is not clear. The fact that they have so far been isolated only in sleep-deprived animals makes it uncertain that they are involved in the normal daily initiation of sleep. Yet they could be part of a series of functional peptide compounds present in the brain (see chap. 9).

Other neurochemical systems are clearly involved in sleep. Hernandez-Peon and his collaborators (1965) have proposed a cholinergic theory of sleep, and have delineated a number of factors or areas in which acetylcholine appears to produce sleep. The problem is that acetylcholine is a transmitter in very many different areas of the brain, and the areas delineated do not appear to be specifically necessary for sleep.

On the basis of present evidence, I believe the serotonin system and the catecholamine systems are most specific to sleep and wakefulness and will be most useful to us in later discussions of sleeping medication.

SLEEP DEPRIVATION

There have been literally hundreds of studies of sleep deprivation in recent years, but overall the results have been somewhat disappointing. Physiologically, a sleep-deprived subject shows a central (brain) hypoarousal, combined, at least in certain stages, with an autonomic nervous system hyperarousal. After several days of sleep deprivation, the waking EEG shifts away from alpha and in the direction of lower frequencies. Pulse and respiratory rates frequently increase. Recovery sleep after a period of sleep deprivation involves in the first hours a great deal of slow-wave sleep (stages 3 and 4) and in subsequent hours or days an increase in D-time.

The psychological effects of sleep deprivation have not always been easy to determine. One obvious fact is that they depend a great deal on social and environmental factors. For instance, a period of sleep deprivation undergone in an army group where such deprivation is seen as a challenge to be overcome has very different effects from sleep deprivation in a 24-hour "marathon group" where the emphasis is on increasing self-awareness and emergence of usually repressed material. There have been many studies investigating what tasks are especially sensitive to sleep deprivation. In general, the conclusion has been that to a small extent the difficulty of a task, but to a far greater extent its length and dullness, make it susceptible to disruption by sleep deprivation. Thus, the only tests that have reliably picked up differences between rested subjects and subjects who have experienced half-a-night's sleep loss are those involving hours of monitoring a TV display, with responses required when certain symbols are seen. Unfortunately, such results can be interpreted as showing merely that a sleep-deprived subject is more likely to fall asleep, since the tasks sensitive to sleep deprivation

are exactly those during which the subject might be expected
to doze off, at least briefly. Although it has been hard to
establish sleep deprivation effects on such objective psychological tests, there is no question that there is a subjective
effect, and this can be measured as an effect on mood.
Various studies involving adjective checklists have found decreases in alertness and vigor and increases in confusion and
fatigue (hardly surprising results!).

Prolonged periods of sleep deprivation have sometimes led
to increasing ego disorganization, hallucinations, and even
delusions. It has been widely assumed that a long enough
period of sleep deprivation would produce a psychosis in
normal subjects, but this cannot be stated with certainty, both
because of obvious ethical considerations in conducting research, and because the occasional subjects who do either
sleep-deprive themselves for long periods, or for that matter
who volunteer for long-term sleep deprivation studies, must
be considered somewhat atypical.

Since the advent of EEG techniques, it has become possible
to deprive persons selectively of D-sleep or of the deeper portions of S-sleep. It is not possible to deprive someone completely of synchronized sleep without producing total sleep
deprivation. Selective D-deprivation produces several unques-
tionable effects (Dement, 1960, and others). First, during the
night when the subject is being awakened at the beginning of
each D-period, he makes an increasing number of attempts
to begin a D-period; thus, while four or five awakenings are
sufficient on the first night, twenty to thirty awakenings are
often required by the fifth, and it is often impossible to continue the study much longer than that. Second, recovery
sleep is usually characterized by greatly increased D-sleep
("rebound" increase).

Psychological effects are less certain. Although it was first
reported that D-deprivation produced disorganization and
would eventually produce psychosis in line with suggestions
made by Freud and others, recent results have not been con-
clusive. It has been possible to differentiate only to a limited

extent the psychological changes produced by D-sleep deprivation from those produced by stage 4 deprivation. One careful study in this area did describe greater physical lethargy in the stage 4-deprived subjects, and more irritability and social difficulties in the D-deprived group (Agnew et al., 1967).

SLEEP REQUIREMENTS

Although the exact functions of sleep are not yet known, and some researchers have proposed that sleep is a habit with no real function at present, most view sleep as having some basic restorative function. Supporting this view is the relative constancy of sleep requirement. Sleep time in young adult humans averages about seven hours and forty-five minutes, and there is surprisingly little variation in this average across differences in culture, temperature, latitude, and so on. For instance, Norwegians above the Arctic Circle, who live under the extreme conditions of the "midnight sun" in summer and the "noon moon" in winter, nonetheless sleep an average of only forty to fifty minutes 'longer in winter.

Therefore, it is likely that a certain amount of sleep is generally required for all humans, although the amount may be hard to determine precisely. In one study a number of normal subjects tried to reduce their sleep per night by fifteen minutes each week and were relatively successful until they reached levels of five to six hours per night, when continuation in the study became very difficult. In one study we attempted to differentiate persons who required a great deal of sleep (over nine hours a day) from those who required very little (less than six hours a day). We found that the long sleepers were generally "worriers" who took things very seriously, had many complaints and worries about themselves and the world, and could be seen as "reprogramming themselves" frequently during the day; while the short sleepers tended to be nonworriers who were relatively "pre-programmed," in other words, had a way of running their lives which satisfied them and which they altered relatively little.

Thus, most people appear to require at least 5 to 6 hours of sleep per 24 hours. Around this minimum there is considerable variation, and sleep requirement may be related to personality or life-style. This is not the place for a detailed discussion of sleep requirements, except to mention that quite obviously a short sleep time without any symptoms or complaints is no reason to take a sleeping pill. I would certainly hope that no one who sleeps five to six hours and feels fine would consider taking medication for this "condition."

THE FUNCTIONS OF SLEEP

After many years of intensive sleep research, I believe most researchers would agree with me that we do not yet totally understand the functions of sleep. One group maintains that sleep presently has no function. These researchers hypothesize that it may have once had a behavioral function, perhaps to keep our early mammalian ancestors out of harm's way for a certain number of hours each day, and may have persisted simply as a sort of habit. Evidence cited in support of this view is that occasionally a person is found who appears to require no sleep—or very little—and also the fact, mentioned above, that several days of sleep deprivation produces very few definable deficiencies in behavior. I do not find this evidence entirely convincing: only one person who slept a few minutes per day has been studied carefully by modern laboratory methods; he had definite psychological and biological abnormalities, and he died within two years of the onset of the short-sleep pattern (see chap. 6). And although it is true that it is difficult to find striking abnormalities on most objective tests after a few days of sleep deprivation, I attribute this fact to the lack of sensitivity of most such tests. Certainly one's subjective state is quite abnormal after sleep deprivation, and this can be quantified by using tests of mood such as adjective checklists.

Another group maintains that it is senseless even to look for the functions of sleep; we should look, rather, for functions of the entire sleep-wakefulness cycle, the W-S-D cycles, or the whole complex of biological cycles.

I believe that sleep does have a biological function, and that we do not sleep simply out of habit. And it seems to me that the functions of the cycles—why the human body contains such a powerful 90-minute oscillator and also a number of oscillators with periods of slightly over 24 hours—are fascinating, but they are quite separate from the question of the functions of sleep.

The activities a mammal performs which are most necessary in order to preserve its own life (feeding, etc.), as well as those necessary for the preservation of the species (mating, preparing a home for the young and caring for them, etc.) all occur during wakefulness. It makes sense from the point of view of optimal adaptation that sleep should play some role in making these important waking activities as efficient and fruitful as possible. My laboratory has performed a great many studies relevant to the functions of sleep, and I have presented conclusions elsewhere (Hartmann, 1973). Figure 4.6 offers a brief summary of these conclusions, but I believe it will be difficult for the reader to follow, and certainly difficult to accept, without reading the context. Basically, I have suggested that S-sleep is a time of anabolism—a time when a synthesis of macromolecules—ribonucleic acids and/ or proteins—is facilitated. I have suggested that D-sleep, which ordinarily follows S-sleep, is a time in which these molecules are used in the brain; it is a time of repair, of reorganization, and of formation of new connections in the brain. Forming new connections involves integrating daytime material which has not been properly integrated or stored during the daytime, and thus also involves the formation of new memory systems. I believe this restoration occurs especially in the cerebral cortex and the brain norepinephrine systems ascending to the cortex; and I further suggest that these systems which are restored during sleep are those required for atten-

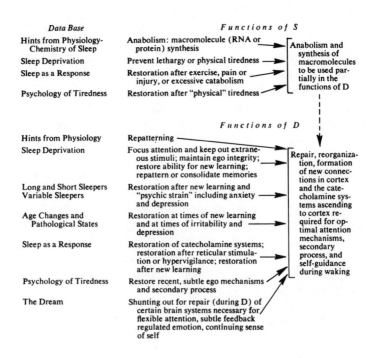

FIGURE 4.6   Functions of Sleep: Summary

tion processes, "secondary process," and overall adaptive self-guidance during waking. Thus, mine is clearly a restorative view of sleep. Obviously a great deal of work still needs to be done in order to confirm or disprove it.

SLEEP IN MENTAL ILLNESS

The possible relationship between sleep disturbance or sleep deprivation and mental illness, and the possible psychological relations between dreaming and psychosis, have led to a large number of laboratory studies investigating sleep in mental illness. Here I can only discuss briefly the questions of whether sleep disturbance or deprivation can actually produce mental illness, whether sleep patterns are altered or disturbed during mental illness, and whether sleep disturbance can have any predictive or prognostic value.

The first question is difficult to answer definitively. Long periods of sleep deprivation have sometimes given rise to transient psychotic symptoms, but only in some people. A healthy high-school student who sleep-deprived himself for a "record" of over 200 hours suffered no psychological changes. Evaluating the role of sleep deprivation in naturally occurring illness is more difficult, but my impression is that few, if any, episodes of psychosis are caused primarily by sleep disturbance or deprivation. However, sleep deprivation may play a part in the vicious cycle preceding a psychotic episode: problems in personal relationships or other aspects of reality produce anxiety, which results in sleeplessness, which in turn leads to increased inability to handle reality, and so on. Sleep disturbance, though not a primary cause, can play a role in initiating a psychotic episode or increasing the severity of existing symptoms. And conversely, obtaining sleep, with or without medication, during the first days of hospitalization can help to reduce the severity of the patient's symptoms.

Sleep patterns during psychiatric illness are now fairly well established. Despite expectations based on associations between dreaming and schizophrenia, the sleep of hospitalized schizophrenic patients studied in the laboratory is relatively normal. During acute episodes, sleep is often disturbed and D-time low, but it is not likely that this is related in any intrinsic manner to the schizophrenic process; it is more probably an effect of extreme anxiety. Some chronic schizophrenic patients show perfectly normal sleep patterns; in others, there is a decrease in slow-wave sleep (stages 3 and 4). We have done a study relating this to the postulated central "hyperarousal" of certain schizophrenic patients.

Mania and depression are associated with unusual sleep patterns. EEG studies have confirmed the very short sleep-time usually found in manic patients: all stages of sleep appear to be reduced to a certain extent, although there is some disagreement between studies. In our investigations, D-sleep was especially reduced, while stage 4-sleep remained close to normal levels.

Sleep is usually abnormal during depression, but several distinct patterns can be described. The most frequent sleep pattern in severe depression involves insomnia—more often difficulty in remaining than in falling asleep. This has been confirmed in laboratory sleep studies. Some depressed patients have frequent awakenings during the night as well as early-morning awakenings, reduced slow-wave sleep-time, and sometimes reduced D-sleep as well. However, other depressed patients have hypersomnia—increased total sleep time without dramatic alterations in sleep stages and usually with increased D-time. In fact, most depressed patients demonstrate an increased tendency to have D-sleep; some have increased D-time, but almost all manifest decreased D-latency, a greater number of D-periods, and increased eye movements during the D-periods. There is no unanimous agreement about the relationship between sleep and depression. Possibly there are two factors: one, an increased need for sleep and D-sleep, present in most or all depression; and two, the additional problem of an inability to remain asleep, present in some severely depressed patients.

Aside from these specific sleep changes in specific illnesses, there is one overall finding that may be very useful to keep in mind and does not depend on sleep laboratory studies. Sleep disturbance (insomnia) is often one of the earliest signs of psychological disturbance. For instance, Detre et al. (1966) studied a group of hospitalized patients who had attempted suicide and tried to determine the earliest warning sign which might have alerted doctors and nurses that something was wrong. Sleep disturbance turned out to be one very early sign. Thus, rapid onset of insomnia is a sign that certainly needs to be investigated since it could signal a serious psychological problem. However, it may have many other causes (see chap. 6).

Sleep disorders can be roughly divided into a number of classes, none of which will be discussed in detail here. First, there are medical and psychosomatic disorders which are *exacerbated* during sleep. For instance, anginal attacks appear to be more frequent during D-sleep, and some studies indicate that extrasystoles (PVBs) are more frequent both during D-sleep and during stage 4 sleep. Second, there are episodic occurrences during sleep. These include enuresis, sleep walking, pavor nocturnus, which occur chiefly during arousals from slow-wave sleep, and tooth-grinding and head-banging which may occur in children during almost any stage of sleep. Third, there is sleep pathology in the stricter sense: "primary sleep disorders". These may involve defects in the sleep-waking mechanisms. Narcolepsy is a special condition characterized by short sleep attacks in the daytime and frequently by cataplexy, sleep paralysis, and hypnagogic hallucinations. Laboratory studies reveal that narcoleptics usually have an abnormally short D-latency at night, and daytime attacks consist of an almost immediate change from waking to D-sleep. Thus, this condition can be seen as a failure of the normal mechanism inhibiting D-periods. Aside from narcolepsy, several other distinct varieties of hypersomnia have been described.

Sleep apnea is a newly discovered condition that can produce the symptoms either of excessive daytime sleepiness or insomnia. In sleep apnea, all-night polygraphic recordings demonstrate many periods when respiration totally ceases; usually this initiates an awakening, respiration resumes, and the process may then repeat itself, sometimes over a hundred times per night. Some cases of apnea may be caused by local pathology—tissue malformation or excessively thick tissues in the pharynx or elsewhere which actually block respiration during sleep. Sometimes the cause is a problem in the brain-stem.

Nocturnal myoclonus is a condition characterized by quick jerks (myoclonic episodes) involving muscles of the legs and sometimes other muscles. Sleep apnea, nocturnal myoclonus, and their treatment will be discussed again in chapter 6.

By far the most common sleep disorder is insomnia. In my view, it can best be seen as a symptom or a final common pathway that can be produced by a number of antecedent causes. Understanding insomnia is obviously central to the concerns of this book, and I shall discuss it in detail in chapter 6.

THE BIOLOGY OF SLEEP
AND THE SLEEPING PILL

We have now briefly surveyed a great deal of basic knowledge about sleep. An interested reader can find more complete information in the References to this chapter. In addition to its general interest, this biological information should obviously be relevant to the investigation of hypnotic medication. First of all, knowledge of the biology of sleep has led to the beginning of a more scientific study of insomnia, and these studies are still in progress (chap. 6): presumably, increased knowledge of insomnia will determine when a sleeping pill is required or when other treatment may be preferable. Also, knowledge of the biology of sleep has brought great advances in our ability to study the effects of any chemical substance on sleep minute by minute on polygraphic records (chap. 5).

Generally, in terms of a discussion of sleeping pills, I believe it is most important to note from the biology discussed that sleep is not simply a lack of wakefulness, nor is it simply a light form of coma or death. The two distinct states of sleep, the recurring cycles, and all the other attendant events I have described here, do not occur in deep coma. Sleep is a unique state. Therefore, in principle, a "good" sleeping pill should

Sleep

not be a poison or an anesthetic taken in small doses, b
should have an action specifically related to the biology c
sleep.

References

Agnew, H. W., Jr.; W. B. Webb; and R. L. Williams. Comparison
of stage four and 1-REM sleep deprivation. *Percept. Motor
Skills* 24 (1967): 851–58.

Aserinsky, E., and N. Kleitman. Regularly occurring periods of eye
motility and concomitant phenomena during sleep. *Science* 118
(1953): 273–74.

———. Two types of ocular motility occurring in sleep. *J. Appl.
Physiol.* 8 (1955): 1–10.

Dement, W. Effect of dream deprivation. *Science* 131 (1960):
1705–07.

Dement, W., and N. Kleitman. Cyclic variations in EEG during
sleep and their relation to eye movements, body motility, and
dreaming. *Electroencephalog. Clin. Neurophysiol.* 9 (1957):
673–90.

Dement, W. C. *Some Must Watch While Some Must Sleep.* San
Francisco: W. H. Freeman, 1974.

Detre, T. Sleep disorder and psychosis. *Can. Psychiat. Assoc. J.* 11
(1966): 5169–77.

Hartmann, E. *The Biology of Dreaming.* Springfield, Ill.: Thomas,
1967.

———. The D-state and norepinephrine-dependent systems. In *Sleep
and Dreaming,* edited by E. Hartmann, pp. 308–28. Boston:
Little, Brown, 1970.

———. *The Functions of Sleep.* New Haven: Yale University Press,
1973.

———. Effects of Psychotropic Drugs on Sleep: The Catecholamines
and Sleep. A Generation of Progress, edited by Morris A. Lipton;
Al. DiMascio; and Keith F. Killiam. In *Psychopharmacology,*
1977.

Hernandez-Peon, R. Central neuro-humoral transmission in sleep
and wakefulness. In Akert, K.; C. Bally; and J. P. Schade, eds.,
Progress in Brain Research, vol. 18: Sleep Mechanisms, pp. 96–
117. Amsterdam: Elsevier, 1965.

Hauri, P. The Sleep Disorders (Current Concepts Series). Kala-
    mazoo, Mich.: Upjohn, 1977.
Hobson, J. A., and R. W. McCarley. Cortical unit activity in sleep
    and waking. *Electroenceph. Clin. Neurophysiol.* 30 (1971): 97–
    112.
———. *Neuronal Activity in Sleep: An Annotated Bibliography.*
    Harvard Medical School, 1977.
Hobson, J. A.; R. W. McCarley; and P. W. Wyzinski. Sleep cycle
    oscillation: reciprocal discharge by two brainstem neuronal
    groups. *Science* 189 (1975): 55–58.
Jouvet, M. Recherches sur les structures nerveuses et les mécanismes
    responsables des différentes phases du sommeil physiologique.
    Arch. Ital. Biol. 100 (1962): 125–206.
———. The role of monoamines and acetylcholine-containing neurons
    in the regulation of the sleep-waking cycle. *Ergeb. Physiol.* 64
    (1972): 166–307.
Kleitman, N. *Sleep and Wakefulness.* Chicago: University of
    Chicago Press, 1963.
Koella, W. P. *Sleep: Its nature and physiological organization.*
    Springfield, Ill.: Thomas, 1967.
Koella, W. P.; A. Feldstein; and J. Czicman. The effect of para-
    chlorophenylalanine on the sleep of cats. *Electroencephalogr.
    Clin. Neurophysiol.* 25 (1968): 481–90.
Kupfer, D.; G. Foster; L. Reich; K. Thompson; and B. Weiss. EEG
    sleep changes as predictors in depression. *Amer. J. Psych.* 133,
    no. 6 (1975): 622–26.
McCarley, R. W., and J. A. Hobson. Neuronal excitability modula-
    tion over the sleep cycle: a structural and mathematical model.
    Science 189 (1976): 58–60.
Mendelson, W. B.; J. C. Gillin; and R. J. Wyatt. *Human Sleep and
    Its Disorders.* New York: Plenum Press, 1977.
Monnier, M.; A. M. Hatt; L. B. Cueni; and G. A. Schoenenberger.
    Humoral transmission of sleep. VI. Purification and assessment
    of a hyponongenic fraction of "sleep dialysate" factor delts. In
    Pflugers Arch. 331 (1974): 257–65.
Monnier, M., and L. Hosli. Dialysis of sleep and waking factors in
    blood of the rabbit. *Science* 146, no. 3645 (1964): 796–98.
Moruzzi, G., and H. Magoun. Brain stem reticular formation and
    activation of the EEG. *Electroenceph. Clin. Neurophysiol.* 1
    (1949): 455–73.

Pappenheimer, J.; T. Miller; and C. Goodrich. Sleep-promoting effect of cerebrospinal fluid from sleep-deprived goats. *Proc. Nat. Acad. Sci. USA.* 58 (1967): 513–17.

Pappenheimer, J. R.; G. Koski; V. Fencl; M. L. Karnovsky; and J. Krueger. Extraction of sleep-promoting factor S from cerebrospinal fluid and from brains of sleep-deprived animals. *J. Neurophysiol.* 38, no. 6 (1975): 1299–1311.

Pompeiano, O. Sleep mechanisms. In *Basic Mechanisms of the Epilepsies,* edited by H. H. Jasper; A. A. Ward, Jr.; and A. Pope, pp. 453–73. Boston: Little, Brown, 1969.

Radulovacki, M. 5-Hydroxyindoleacetic acid in cerebrospinal fluid: Measurements in wakefulness, slow-wave and paradoxical sleep. *Brain Research* 50, no. 2 (1973): 484–88. Reviewed in *Sleep Research* 3 (1974): 251.

Roffwarg, H.; J. Muzio; and W. Dement. Ontogenetic development of human sleep-dream cycle. *Science* 152 (1966): 604–19.

Webb, W. *Sleep The Gentle Tyrant.* Englewood Cliffs, N.J.: Prentice-Hall, 1975.

Wilkinson, R. T. Sleep deprivation: Performance tests for partial and selective sleep deprivation. *Prog. Clin. Psychol.* 8 (1968): 28–43.

Williams, H. L.; A. Lubin.; and J. J. Goodnow. Impaired performance with acute sleep loss. *Psychol. Monogr. General and Applied* 73 (1959): 1–26.

Williams, R. L.; T. Karacan; and C. J. Hursch. *EEG of Human Sleep: Clinical Applications.* New York: John Wiley & Sons, 1974.

———. *Pharmacology of Sleep.* New York: John Wiley & Sons, 1976.

Zarcone, V.; G. Gulevich; T. Pivik; and W. Dement. Partial REM phase deprivation and schizophrenia. *Arch. Gen. Psychiat.* 18 (1968): 194–202.

5

The Effect of Sleeping Pills on Sleep

The material reviewed in the last chapter makes it obvious that modern all-night polygraphic sleep recordings afford us an excellent way to determine with great precision the effect of drugs or other independent variables on sleep patterns. Although, as I mentioned, such studies cannot totally be substituted for knowledge of the subjective effects of a drug, we are now in a position to study not only subjective effect or length of sleep as reported by an observer: we can determine the effects of a medication on time taken to fall asleep and to reach the various normal stages of sleep; time spent in the two major states and the four stages of sleep; the exact number of awakenings and time spent in each awakening; the length of time spent in each stage of sleep; and also many more measures, such as the number of eye movements during D-periods, the number of sleep spindles during S-sleep, and other determinations that may sometimes be of interest.

We can and should whenever possible study the effect of drugs upon all the variables above, not only when the drug is first administered for a single night, but also its effects after continuing or long-term administration and after drug withdrawal.

The richness of the data thus obtained can be useful in many ways. For instance, I have frequently emphasized that all-night polygraphic sleep studies are one of the few methods we have for studying long-term alterations of brain function after medication or after other stimuli or illnesses that can affect the brain; and these continuous recordings appear to be an especially sensitive measure. Thus, long-term sleep recordings are of great value in a number of different areas aside from the evaluation of sleeping medications. In fact, at last count there were over one thousand separate studies investigating the effects of various drugs or other forms of stimuli on recorded sleep. For our present purposes, however, I shall examine only studies involving the effects of drugs upon sleep patterns, and of these I shall concentrate on studies investigating the effects of sleeping pills or drugs that can be defined in some sense as "hypnotic medication." Even this is no small task, since there are now several hundred such studies.

The bulk of the hard data on this topic is contained in the long table at the end of this chapter (table 5.1) and in Appendices A and B. Appendix A reproduces several actual laboratory studies investigating the effects of long-term administration and withdrawal of several important drugs upon laboratory-recorded sleep. Appendix B presents a clinical study comparing the effects of two sleeping medications and placebo in a clinical outpatient population. I hope that the reader interested either in these specific results or in the methodology involved in sleep research studies will examine the material in these appendixes.

What I shall do here is summarize in a few paragraphs the results presented extensively in table 5.1, as well as the data discussed more intensively in Appendices A and B; I shall then offer a series of comments and suggestions for future studies and evaluations of sleeping medications.

SUMMARY OF RESULTS

Table 5.1 presents the results of several hundred sleep laboratory studies involving hypnotic agents.* It includes studies done through 1975 involving all

* This table is reprinted, including minor alterations, with permission, from D. Kay, A. Blackburn, J. Buckingham, and I. Karacan, "Human Pharmacology of Sleep," in *Pharmacology of Sleep*, ed. R. Williams and I. Karacan (New York: John Wiley & Sons, 1976).

groups of drugs generally available as hypnotics but does not include studies of l-tryptophan and related natural food substances; l-tryptophan will be discussed in chapter 11. Studies in normal subjects, in insomniacs, and in certain other special groups such as depressed patients are included.

The barbiturates, probably the most widely used hypnotic agents in the world, are listed first in the table, and have been the most widely studied group until the past few years. Despite a large number of studies listed, very few have investigated more than one dose level, and likewise few have studied long-term administration and withdrawal, so our overall knowledge is still rather limited; but a few conclusions readily emerge. At the usual clinical doses, the barbiturates do generally reduce sleep latency, and sometimes increase sleep time, especially when insomniac patients are studied. However, they also clearly produce distortions in normal sleep patterns. The most striking effect, found in every case, is that D-sleep (REM sleep) is reduced by all the barbiturates. This effect continues on long-term administration, though there is a gradual return toward baseline, so that after some weeks D-time returns to levels only somewhat below normal. However, an abnormality is clearly present, which is most easily demonstrable when drug administration is discontinued: there is a sudden and pronounced increase in D-time upon drug withdrawal. Some qualitative effects are also produced by the barbiturates, especially an increase in fast-wave EEG activity.

The benzodiazepines have become the most widely used group of hypnotics and are represented by numerous studies in table 5.1. In general, these drugs, too, reduce sleep latency and increase sleep time, and this is noted especially when insomniacs rather than normal subjects are studied. The benzodiazepines also produce considerable changes in the stages of sleep, although this fact is not always evident on the first night of drug administration and was thus missed in early studies involving only one night. Starting with the second or third night, and continuing on long-term administration, the benzodiazepines produce clear-cut reductions in D-sleep and in stage 4—the deepest portion of S-sleep. The reductions in D-sleep and stage 4 sleep (sometimes also stage 3) continue on chronic administration and appear to return gradually to normal after discontinuation, without any very dramatic rebounds in the other direction. The benzodiazepines also produce an interesting qualitative change in sleep records, of unknown significance: the number of sleep spindles—the characteristic 12 to 14 per-second activity of stage 2 sleep—is greatly increased. Many other hypnotic medications also produce a slight increase in this measure.

Chloral hydrate has been the subject of a number of studies. It is interesting that, in contrast to the drug groups mentioned above, chloral hydrate in the usual clinical doses—ranging from 500 mg through 1500 mg at bedtime—produces very little change or distortion of normal sleep patterns. Questions have been raised as to whether chloral hydrate at the usual doses actually has hypnotic effects, but the studies listed in the table, although there are not many, tend to support its effectiveness. The only study involving insomniac patients shows that 1000 mg of chloral hydrate reduced sleep latency, and one of the more solid studies investigating healthy normal controls also showed a significant increase in sleep time and a decrease in sleep latency (even though it is normally very difficult to demonstrate such effects in normal subjects, since they sleep relatively well on placebo).

Glutethimide turns out to be somewhat similar to the barbiturates in terms of its effect on sleep recordings, but its effect at the usual doses is weaker. It is barely effective or not clearly effective in inducing sleep, but it does clearly reduce D-time and increase D-latency. Methaqualone and methyprylon similarly reduce D-time and increase D-latency. These studies at least suggest usefulness in inducing sleep and reducing sleep latency.

The antihistamines—especially diphenhydramine and methapyrilene—also tend to reduce D-time. The studies listed in table 5.1 showed no clear improvement in sleep patterns, but several recent studies do suggest that the antihistamines have at least minimal sleep-reducing effects.

In general, then, one can conclude from the table that most hypnotic medications are effective—though sometimes minimally effective—in the sense that they reduce sleep latency or waking time when first administered and when studied in insomniac patients. Even in the cases where improved sleep does occur, however, there is evidence that these improvements are not maintained through long-term use (52, 53, 55). For some medications, such as the antihistamines, even results on the first night of administration are not clear-cut. Additional work is required to demonstrate a distinct superiority over placebo. What is most evident from the table is the fact that most or all hypnotic medications investigated produced a distortion of normal sleep patterns—most frequently a reduction in D-sleep (REM sleep), often accompanied by an increase in D-latency and a decrease in the number of eye movements when these are counted. In the case of the benzodiazepines, there is in addition a definite reduction in stage 4 sleep. Thus the distortions in normal physiological sleep patterns are the clearest findings of these laboratory studies.

COMMENTS AND CONCERNS

Table 5.1 is far more complete and thorough than most such tabulations, and I have borrowed it purposely for that reason. It even includes some drugs among the benzodiazepines that are usually sold as tranquilizers rather than sleeping pills. It is nonetheless interesting that many substances with clear sleep-inducing properties do not appear in this table or in other tables of hypnotics—nor, for that matter, in textbook chapters on hypnotic medication. I believe the problem is that we are too ready to use the marketplace for definitional criteria and to call a "hypnotic medication" simply whatever is currently sold as such. For instance, the opiates—morphine and related substances—are not included at all, even though we know that these are among the oldest sleeping pills. Presumably they do not appear because they are now usually listed as analgesics; also, the fact that they are addictive and widely abused has made it legally impossible to prescribe or purchase them as sleeping pills, at least in the United States.

Other substances, such as the phenothiazines and other dopamine receptor blockers, are not mentioned as sleeping pills because their chief action is antipsychotic. Some substances, such as the amino acid l-tryptophan, which has been shown to have clear sleep-inducing properties in laboratory studies (chap. 10), presumably are not included because they are not currently marketed as sleeping pills in the United States. It is somewhat ironic that these drugs are not included in such a complete and excellent review of hypnotics since, as we shall see later, these three groups of substances may turn out to be more logical and reasonable as sleeping pills than any others. The effects of the best-known dopamine blocker, chlorpromazine, are presented in detail in Appendix A. All three groups are discussed as possible sleeping pills in chapter 9.

I might mention here some other substances that are occasionally used to produce sleep but do not appear in tables or chapters on hypnotic medication: alcohol and marijuana or hashish. Neither alcohol nor marijuana has been found to be particularly effective in inducing or maintaining sleep in laboratory studies; in fact, there are many studies demonstrating that alcohol taken in large doses, or continuously, has extremely disruptive effects on sleep. Nonetheless, the pattern of brain effects produced by alcohol—including early reduction of tension or anxiety when taken in small doses—makes it useful to some individuals as a sleeping pill. Some persons find the relaxing effects of marijuana helpful for sleep induction, while others experience chiefly stimulating effects.

A related conclusion that emerges from these data is one already suggested in an earlier chapter. It is amazing how many drugs of widely differing chemical structure are listed and are effective as hypnotic agents. It is clear that many of these agents would appear in other tables as well: the barbiturates and some of the others function as anesthetic agents as well as hypnotics. The benzodiazepines are used as antianxiety agents in the daytime; the antihistamines are chiefly taken for their ability to counter the effects of histamine and thus reduce allergic reactions. Obviously, sleeping pills are a very heterogeneous group of substances, with little in common except that they produce general depression of the central nervous system. There is little reason to believe that most of these agents have any action relating to normal sleep, and in fact we have seen that many of them produce abnormal or distorted sleep recordings.

It is somewhat disturbing that we are so willing to accept all these various substances as hypnotic agents or sleeping pills simply because they are sold as such and because, in a behavioral sense, they "put people to sleep," even though the "sleep" they produce does not look like physiologically normal sleep. Should we not logically include other ways of "putting people to sleep," such as chloroform, ether, various poisons, or, for that matter, a sharp blow to the head?

METHODOLOGY AND THOUGHTS FOR FUTURE DRUG STUDIES

Several methodological problems emerge in reviewing these studies (table 5.1). The field of laboratory sleep research is a young one, and understandably we have all tried to accomplish a great deal—perhaps too much—with limited resources. Many of the studies reviewed, including some of my own, attempt to make a contribution both to the basic pharmacology of sleep and to testing the efficacy of sleeping pills. In a preliminary study when a drug is first being investigated, these two aims may be compatible, but in terms of good study design and eventual definitive results, the two aims are very different.

If one wishes to make a contribution to the pharmacology of sleep—for instance, to investigate what effect a certain medication which alters brain chemistry will have upon D-sleep time, stage 4 time, etc.—one must clearly study *normal subjects.* One cannot draw any conclusions, for instance, from insomniac patients whose baseline sleep involves very abnormal amounts of these stages. (For instance, if insomniac patients have very low amounts of stage X before medication, and when taking drug A are found to sleep longer and better and to have increased stage X, one cannot conclude that drug A increases stage X. The increased stage X may merely be an indication that sleep is improved or lengthened; drug A may well have no effect on stage X in normal subjects.)

On the other hand, if one wishes to test the efficacy of a medication as a possible sleeping pill, normal sleepers are not appropriate subjects. For instance, a medication may in fact be able to produce definite decreases in sleep latency (time taken to fall asleep) in insomniacs or persons with long sleep latencies, but it may be entirely impossible to demonstrate this effect in a group of normal subjects whose sleep latency ordinarily is only five minutes. Thus, in testing directly the efficacy of a hypnotic medication, one must use as subjects a group of patients (insomniacs) representing those who will take the medication clinically.

We can now begin to see that development and testing of a potential new sleeping pill is a complex endeavor. At the minimum, a potential sleeping pill must first be tested on both short-term and long-term bases in animals to establish toxicity, safety, and a rough estimate of a human dose. If the drug appears to be safe for animals, and some animal studies suggest sleep-inducing properties, it can then be tested very cautiously on a few human subjects to establish safety in man and to estimate possible doses for further studies. The effects of a single administration on a single night of sleep at various doses must be investigated in order to obtain a dose-response curve and to choose one or two probably effective doses.

After all of this has been accomplished, it is possible to examine pharmacological effects: short-term effects, long-term effects, and withdrawal effects, as in the studies presented in Appendix A. Such studies are not truly studies of efficacy in improving sleep patterns, but rather pharmacological investigations of alterations in brain function and activity by one of the most sensitive methods known. Then studies of efficacy must be done involving populations of insomniac patients likely to use the hypnotic. Ideally, studies of efficacy should include (1) a small group (perhaps 1 to 12 subjects studied intensively in the laboratory so that exact measures of sleep latency, changes in waking time, and so on, can be detected, both when the drug is first given, later during administration, and upon withdrawal; and (2) larger studies with perhaps 50 to 200 subjects but not employing sleep laboratory procedures, since their cost would be prohibitive. The second type of study would evaluate sleep through subjective questionnaires, doctor's reports, and so on (see Appendix B), or in the case of hospitalized patients, on the basis of nighttime observation by nurses. Objective sleep recordings are of obvious importance, but I think it essential that we not omit subjective reports—how the patient actually feels he has slept and how he feels in the morning. Even in ordinary laboratory sleep studies, it is useful to obtain a careful subjective report (by questionnaire or interview) on whether the patient has felt better or worse, or has felt his functioning to have been better or worse (and in what ways) since taking medication.

Insofar as possible, the studies should include not only a description of how the patient feels the next morning, but some measure of how he functions during the day after taking medication, or during the day after he has been taking the medication for a few weeks. This is not always easy, since adequate laboratory tests of human functioning are complicated, time-consuming, and probably not very representative of actual human work and social interactions. A recent review by Bixler et al. (1975) summarizes work done on the effects of hypnotic drugs on daytime performance. The most salient conclusion is that too little work has been done in this area; the last few years have seen a bare beginning of efforts to evaluate the effects of hypnotic medication on various behavior the next day. Tasks have included—among others—reaction time, finger-tapping rate, card-sorting, "shooting gallery," "tracking," various arithmetic and "reasoning" tests, and various tests of vigilance.

The results are not easy to compare or summarize, since different labs use different tests administered at different times of day to different subject groups.* So all the data must be considered as preliminary. To my mind, no catastrophic findings emerge but the data do give some cause for concern. One half or more of the studies could find no significant differences between various hypnotic drugs and placebo, whereas the other third or half did find some differences in performance—differences statistically significant though not huge in magnitude. The differences were almost always in the direction of better performance after placebo than after drug. Thus, the sense of feeling "drugged" or "groggy" the morning after taking a sleeping pill, as described by many users, is not purely a subjective feeling: it is reflected, to a certain extent, in poor performance. Obviously this area requires further study. After all this testing, it would also be useful to establish possible interactions between the new drug and other commonly ingested substances such as alcohol, caffeine, nicotine, and marijuana. These studies need not be exhaustive, but some information is necessary.

* Most of these studies contain an especially troublesome methodological problem related to the above discussion about when normal subjects or insomniacs are most appropriate for study. The subjects tested, after placebo and after drug, were often insomniac patients. This makes sense clinically (as discussed) if such studies are part of a clinical evaluation of safety and efficacy in a population likely to use the drug. However, such studies cannot answer the basic pharmacological question of whether the drug itself had an effect on behavior the next day, since drug effects are confounded by "sleep effects." Let us say that insomniacs taking drug A performed as well the next morning as when taking a placebo. This might mean the drug has no effect on performance, or it might mean that the drug produced poor performance but at the same time the improved sleep with the drug produced improved performance, and the two effects more or less canceled out. To answer this, one has to know the effect on the performance of normal subjects.

Adequate and complete guidelines for development and testing of hypnotic medication are not yet available, although several attempts already exist and several sets of rough guidelines have been drawn up by the Food and Drug Administration. I am a member of a group called the Drug Research Advisory Council of the Association for the Psychophysiological Study of Sleep (APSS), which is trying to formulate comprehensive guidelines for testing sleeping pills.

KEY TO ABBREVIATIONS IN TABLE 5.1

a hs	Before bedtime		or placebo nights (protocol description)
act.	Activity		
AM	Morning	PCPA	*p*-Chlorophenylalanine
B	Baseline or baseline night(s)	per.	Period(s)
BAC	Blood level alcohol	PIP	Phasic integrated potentials
bid	Twice daily	PM	Afternoon or evening
bw	Body weight	*po*	Per os (by mouth)
C	Chronic (study type)	Pt	Patient(s)
cc	Cubic centimeter	q	Every (e.g., q 2 hr = every 2 hours)
CSF	Cerebrospinal fluid		
D	Drug or drug night(s)	*qid*	Four times daily
da	Day(s)	R	Recovery or recovery night(s)
den.	Density	REM	Rapid eye movement
DE	Dose–Effect study (study type)	REMS	REM sleep (same as D-sleep)
		S	Sleep
DI	Interval between drug administrations	Ss	Subjects
		sc	Subcutaneous
EMG	Electromyogram	SS	Sleep samples
EDA	Electrodermal activity	ST	Short-term (study type)
f	Female(s)	SW	Slow-wave
GH	Growth hormone	SWS	Slow-wave sleep
gm	Gram(s)	*tid*	Three times daily
H	Habituation or habituation night(s)	vs	Versus
		W	Withdrawal or withdrawal night(s)
hr	Hour(s)		
hs	Bedtime	wk	Week(s)
HVA	Homovanillic acid	yr	Year(s)
Hy	Healthy	5-HIAA	5-Hydroxyindoleacetic acid
Hz	Cycles per second	0	Stage awake
im	Intramuscular	1	Stage 1 sleep
iv	Intravenous	2	Stage 2 sleep
lat.	Latency	3	Stage 3 sleep
M	Movements	4	Stage 4 sleep
m	Male(s)	$\leq$	Up to
MBDS	Minimal brain dysfunction syndrome	$\geq$	At least
		$<$	Less than
mg	Milligram(s)	$>$	Greater than
MHPG	3-Methoxy-4-hydroxyphenyl-glycol	$\times$	Times
		#	Number
min	Minute(s)	*	Definitive study (study type)
ml	Milliliters	%	Percent or percentage
mo	Month(s)	↑	Increase
N	Number of subjects; or noon	↓	Decrease
NREMS	Non-REM sleep stages (S-sleep)	~	Approximately
NSC	No significant changes	⊙ (period)	Discontinuous nights (in protocol description)
nt	Night(s)		
oz	Ounce(s)	?	Not stated or unclear in published material
P	Pilot (study type); or placebo		

TABLE 5.1: The Effect of Sedative–Hypnotic Drugs on Laboratory Recorded Sleep

DRUG Investigators	Study Type	Subjects	Drug Regimen	Effects on Sleep Parameters — REMS	NREMS	Other	Protocol and Comments
AMOBARBITAL Oswald & Priest, 1965	P	N = 2 Hy	400 mg 600 }	↓ REMS (W ↑) ↑ REMS lat. (W ↓)		↑ Fast act.	5B 9D(400 mg) 9D(600 mg) 6wkW SS: intermittent
Evans & Lewis, 1968	P	N = 2 Hy	400 mg 30 min *a hs*	↓ REMS (tolerance developed)			6B 14D$_1$ 2R 5D$_2$ 45R SS: intermittent D$_{1 \text{ and } 2}$: amobarbital, chlorpromazine DI: 3 da
Evans et al, 1968	P	N = 2 Hy f	200 mg 11 PM	↓ REMS ↑ REMS lat.		↑ S time ↓ S lat.	1H 6wkB 26D 14W SS: intermittent, 1H, 5-6B, 11D, 8W
Haider, 1969	DE	N = 6 Hy	200 mg	↓ REMS	→ 1 ↓ 2	↓ S lat. → M	1H.1P.1D.1P SS: weekly Analyzed thirds of nt
Haider & Oswald, 1971	DE (*200 mg)	N = 6 Hy m	200 mg (N = 6) 400 mg (N = 3)	200 mg: ↓ REMS ↑ REMS lat.		200 mg: ↓ S lat. → Shifts to 0 or 1 → M → Spontaneous EDA	1HP.[1D(200 mg),1D(200 mg)],1P. IP, in balanced order] 1 mo off [1D(200 mg),1D(200 mg). IP,IP, in balanced order]. 1D(400 mg),1D(400 mg) SS: weekly 400 mg: results in same direction as for 200 mg but not analyzed statistically
Perkins & Hinton, 1974	DE	N = 12 Pt, neurotic insomniacs 2 m, 10 f, 20–60 yr	130 mg 11 PM 200 mg 11 PM }		↑ 1 ↑ 2	↑ S time	2HD$_1$,[2D$_2$ (different doses) 3D$_3$ (different doses) IP, in Latin square design] SS consecutive D$_{1-3}$: triclofos, amobarbital, chlordiazepoxide DI: ≥1 da

TABLE 5.1 (continued)

DRUG Investigators	Study Type	Subjects	Drug Regimen	Effects on Sleep Parameters			Protocol and Comments
				REMS	NREMS	Other	
AMOBARBITAL (cont.) Fujii, 1973 Cf. Okuma et al., 1975	ST	N = 4 Hy m	200 mg 1 hr *a hs*	↓ REMS (R ↑) ↓ REM den. ↓ Total REM act.	↑ 2 ↓ 3 + 4	↓ S lat.	3BP 3D 2RP; SS: consecutive; 6 other D, same protocol: bromazepam, flurazepam, medazepam, nitrazepam, imipramine, chlorpromazine; DI: ≥10 da; English summary
Feinberg et al., 1974	ST	N = 4 Hy	32 mg *bid* (8 AM, 1 PM) 32 mg *tid* (8 AM, 1 PM, 5 PM)	↓ REMS ↓ REM den.			4B 2D(64 mg)/4D(96 mg) 3R; SS: ?
Firth, 1974	ST°	N = 8 Hy	200 mg *hs* 400 mg *hs*	↓ REM den.			1wkBP 1wkD(200 mg) 1wkD(400 mg) 1wkR, double-blind; SS: 1–2BP, 1–2D(800 mg), 1–2D (400 mg), 1–2R; Several nt, awakenings for dream reports; Only REM data reported
Hata, 1975	ST	N = 4 Hy	200 mg	↓ REMS ↓ REM den. ↓ total REM act.			3B 3D 2RP; SS: consecutive; 3 other D, same protocol: nitrazepam, imipramine, chlorpromazine; DI: ≥10 da; Only REMS parameters reported; English summary

TABLE 5.1 (continued)

DRUG Investigators	Study Type	Subjects	Drug Regimen	Effects on Sleep Parameters			Protocol and Comments
				REMS	NREMS	Other	
AMOBARBITAL (cont.) Ogunremi et al., 1973	C	N = 8 Hy m	≤25 mg tid, 200 mg hs (N = 4) ≤50 mg tid, 400 mg hs (N = 4)	↑ REMS (W ↑)	(W ↑ SWS)	↓ Shifts to 0 or 1	3wkBP 1wkD(low) 4wkD(high) 3wkWP SS: intermittent, 1BP, 1D(low), D1–D7(high), D21–D28(high), WP1–WP4, WP14–WP21 1 other D, same protocol: benzoctamine Blood samples for GH and corticosteroid levels taken via catheter on nt other than S data nt
HEPTOBARBITAL Oswald et al., 1963	ST*	N = 6 Pt, depressed 2 m, 4 f, 33–67 yr N = 6 Hy	400 mg hs	N = 12: ↓ REMS	N = 12: →0 →1 Pt vs Hy: →0 →2 →4	N = 12: ↓ Stage shifts ↓M Pt vs Hy: ↑M	1H (2P 2D, in balanced order) SS: consecutive
PENTOBARBITAL Williams et al., 1968	P	N = ?	200 mg hs	↓ REMS (W ↑ REMS)	↑4 4 returned		Protocol? 10yrD 2moW
Kales et al., 1968	P	N = 1 Pt, addict m, 23 yr	1000 mg/da				SS: ?BD after 10 yr D, intermittent W Abstract

TABLE 5.1 (*continued*)

DRUG / Investigators	Study Type	Subjects	Drug Regimen	REMS	NREMS	Other	Protocol and Comments
PENTOBARBITAL (cont.) Kales et al., 1968	P	$N = 2$	100 mg hs (N = 1) 200 mg hs (N = 1)	↓ REMS (R ↑) ↑ REMS lat. (R ↓)			3HBP 3D 2RP SS: consecutive
Brazier & Beecher, 1952 Cf. Brazier, 1966	DE°	$N = 9$	90 mg		↑ SW act.	↓ M	1D.1P SS: weekly 3 hr data analyzed from each nt
Rechtschaffen & Maron, 1964	DE	$N = 7$ Hy	100 mg hs				$1D_1,1D_2$, in balanced order SS: both nt $D_{1\ and\ 2}$: pentobarbital, pentobarbital + d-amphetamine DI: ≥ 2 da
Baekeland, 1967°	DE°	$N = 15$ Hy	100 mg	↓ REMS ↑ REMS lat. ↓ REM den.		↓ S lat. → M	$(1D_1,1D_1)$ $(1D_2,1D_2)$, in balanced order SS: weekly $D_{1\ and\ 2}$: pentobarbital, pentobarbital + d-amphetamine
Hartmann, 1968	DE°	$N = 7$ Hy	100 mg 30 min a hs	↓ REMS		↔ S time ↓ S lat.	$2H \geq 4B$ $(1D_1,1D_2,1D_2,1D_3, 1D_4,1D_4,1P$, in random order) SS: weekly D_{1-4}: pentobarbital, amitriptyline, chlordiazepoxide, flurazepam DI: 1 wk
Williams & Agnew, 1969	DE	$N = 27$ Hy m	100 mg 15 min a hs (N = 18) 200 mg 15 min a hs (N = 9)	↓ REMS	↑2		$1P.1D_1,1D_2$, in random order SS: all D and P Other D: meprobamate DI: 2 da 2 studies of 100 mg (N = 9 for each) and 1 study of 200 mg, all with same protocol

77

TABLE 5.1 (*continued*)

DRUG Investigators	Study Type	Subjects	Drug Regimen	Effects on Sleep Parameters			Protocol and Comments
				REMS	NREMS	Other	
PENTOBARBITAL (cont.) Kay et al., 1972	DE°	N = 8 Pt, nondependent opiate addicts m	75 mg/70 kg bw 30 min a *hs* 150 mg/70 kg bw 30 min a *hs* 300 mg/70 kg bw 30 min a *hs*	↓ REMS ↑ REMS lat. ↑ # REMS per. ↓ REMS per. length ↓ REM den.	↑ 2 ↑ Spindle burst act.	↓ M ↓ EMG artifact	4H 3D₁ (different doses) 1P, 3D₂ (different doses) IP, single-blind, in randomized crossover design SS: weekly Other D: morphine DI: 1 wk
Borenstein & Cujo, 1974	ST	N = 3 Pt, insomniacs N = 3, good sleepers	100 mg a *hs*	↓ REMS (R ↑) ↑ REMS lat.		↓ # Awakenings (R ↑) Pt only: ↑ S time	3+H 4B 1D 8R SS: 4B, 1D, R3, R8 3 other D, same protocol: diazepam, lorazepam, nitrazepam DI: ?
Borenstein & Cujo, 1974	ST	N = 3 Pt, insomniacs N = 3, good sleepers	100 mg a *hs*	↓ REMS (R ↑) ↑ REMS lat.		↓ # Awakenings (R ↑) Pt only: ↑ S time	3+H 4B 8D 8R SS: 4B, D3, D8, R3, R8 3 other D, same protocol: diazepam, lorazepam, nitrazepam DI: ?
Kales et al., 1970	ST	N = 4	100 mg	↓ REMS (R ↑)	→ 0 ↓ 4		2H 1BP 3D 2BP SS: consecutive
Gaillard & Aubert, 1975	ST	N = 4 Hy	0.61 mg/kg bw 20 min a *hs* 1.83 mg/kg bw 20 min a *hs*	↓ REMS	↑ 2 ↑ Spindle act.	↑ M	1D(low) 1D(high) IR SS: consecutive 2 other D (oxazepam, thioridazine), same protocol except 1H and 2BP preceded thioridazine DI: 4 wk

78

TABLE 5.1 (continued)

DRUG Investigators	Study Type	Subjects	Drug Regimen	Effects on Sleep Parameters REMS	NREMS	Other	Protocol and Comments
PENTOBARBITAL (cont.) Kales et al., 1974	C	N = 3 Pt, insomniacs taking D; N = 10 Pt, insomniac controls	300–400 mg/nt	↓ REMS	↑2 No SWS		1+yrD; SS: 2–3 nt after 1+yrD; Comparison: Pt on D vs Pt controls
Kales et al., 1975	C	N = 4 Pt, insomniacs	100 mg		↓0 ↓ SWS	↑ # Awakenings	1P 3BP 4wkD 2+wkW; SS: 3 consecutive nt intermittently
PHENOBARBITAL Itil, 1969	P	N = 1 Pt, schizophrenic m, 28 yr	250 mg		↓ 0	↓ S lat. ↓ # Awakenings	1D
Saletu & Itil, 1973	P	N = 1 Pt, enuretic sleepwalker f, 52 yr	100 mg hs	↓ REMS	↑2 ↑3 + 4	↓ S lat.	2H 1B.1D$_1$,1D$_2$,1D$_3$,1D$_4$; SS: all H, B and D nt; D$_{1-4}$: diazepam, flurazepam, phenobarbital, diphenylhydantoin; DI: 4 da
Lester & Guerrero-Figueroa, 1966	DE	N = 6 Hy	120 mg (N = 4); 240 mg (N = 2)		↑4	↑ 18–26 Hz act.	1H.1B.1B 1D$_1$(120 mg) 1D$_1$(240 mg) 1D$_2$,1D$_3$,1D$_4$,1B; SS: weekly; D$_{1-4}$: phenobarbital, alpha chloralose, thiopental, chlorpromazine; DI: 1 wk

TABLE 5.1 (*continued*)

DRUG Investigators	Study Type	Subjects	Drug Regimen	Effects on Sleep Parameters			Protocol and Comments
				REMS	NREMS	Other	
PHENOBARBITAL (cont.) Takahashi et al., 1968	DE	N = 3 Hy	100 mg 30 min *a hs*			↑ Plasma GH peaks	1–2B $1D_1,1D_2, \ldots .1D_6$ SS: all B and D D_{1-6}: imipramine, chlorpromazine, phenobarbital, diphenylhydantoin, chlordiazepoxide, isocarboxid (sequence?) DI: 1 wk–5 mo GH also studied
Feinberg et al., 1969 Cf. Feinberg et al., 1974	ST	N = 6 Pt, severely ill schizophrenics (3) or sociopathic character disorder (3)	200 mg 40 min *a hs*	↓ REMS ↓ REM den.	→ 0 → 1 ↓ 4	↓ # Awakenings → M	$5BP.4–5D_1.4–5RP.4–5D_2.4–5RP$ SS: consecutive wk nt $D_{1\ and\ 2}$: phenobarbital, chlorpromazine in 4 Pt, reverse order in 2 Pt DI: 9–10 da
Zung, 1973	ST	N = 5 Hy 3m, 2 f, 20–45 yr	100 mg *a hs*				$4B.2D_1\ 2RP.2D_2$ SS: 2–4 consecutive nt of 3 consecutive wk $D_{1\ and\ 2}$: phenobarbital, triclofos DI: 6 da
SECOBARBITAL Williams, 1954	DE	N = 15	100 mg			↓ S lat. ↑ 18–30 Hz act.	Protocol? 1 other D: methylparafynol for comparison

TABLE 5.1 (continued)

DRUG Investigators	Study Type	Subjects	Drug Regimen	Effects on Sleep Parameters			Protocol and Comments
				REMS	NREMS	Other	
SECOBARBITAL (cont.) Edsjö & Dureman, 1968	DE°	$N = 12$ Hy	200 mg		→0 →1 →2	↓ S lat. → Stage shifts	Protocol? (double-blind, random sequence of D and P) SS: 3+ nt 3 other D: aprobarbital + vinbarbital, nealbarbital, nealbarbital + secobarbital DI: 3+ da English summary
Lehmann & Ban, 1968	DE°	$N = 10$ Hy 4 m, 6 f, 19–25 yr	100 mg	↓ REMS			1B.($1D_1,1D_2,1D_3,1D_4,1P$, in Latin square design) SS: weekly D_{1-4}: secobarbital, nitrazepam, chloral hydrate, chlorprothixene DI: 1 wk
Lester et al., 1968	DE°	$N = 14$ Hy m, 20–24 yr	200 mg 30 min a hs	↓ REMS ↓ REM den.	↑2 →↓ Spindle act.	↓ M ↑ Fast act.	≥3BP.1D 1R.1BP, double-blind SS: weekly, except consecutive D and R
Lester, 1960	DE	$N = 5$ 3 m, 2 f	50 mg 100 mg }	NSC	NSC	NSC	1H.[$1P.1D_1$(50 mg).$1D_1$(100 mg). $1D_2$(50 mg).$1D_2$(100 mg), in Latin square design] SS: all D and P $D_{1 \text{ and } 2}$: secobarbital, thalidomide DI: ?

81

TABLE 5.1 (continued)

DRUG Investigators	Study Type	Subjects	Drug Regimen	Effects on Sleep Parameters			Protocol and Comments
				REMS	NREMS	Other	
SECOBARBITAL (cont.) Allnut & O'Connor, 1971	DE°	N = 8 Hy	100 mg		↑ 2	↑ S time ↓ S lat.	1B.1D$_1$,1P.1D$_2$,1P.1D$_3$,1B.1D$_1$, double-blind, balanced design, no consecutive active D SS: every other nt Other D: nitrazepam DI: 4 da
Feinberg et al., 1974	ST	N = 4 Hy	100–200 mg	↓ REMS ↓ REM den.			4B 7–8D 3R SS: ?
NEALBARBITAL Edsjö & Dureman, 1968	DE°	N = 12 Hy	200 mg				Protocol? (double-blind, random sequence of D and P) SS: 3+ nt 3 other D: secobarbital . . . DI: 3+ da English summary
THIOPENTAL Lester & Guerrero-Figueroa, 1966	DE	N = 4 Hy	300 mg iv	↓ REMS ↑ REMS lat.	↑ 4	↑ S time	1H.1B.1B.1D$_1$(120 mg),1D$_1$(240 mg),1D$_2$,1D$_3$,1D$_4$.1B SS: weekly D$_{1-2}$: phenobarbital, alpha chloralose, thiopental, chlorpromazine DI: 1 wk
COMBINATION: AMOBARBITAL + SECOBARBITAL (TUINAL®) Evans et al., 1968	P	N = 1 m	300 mg amobarbital +300 mg secobarbital/da	↓ REMS (W ↑)		(W ↓ S time) (W ↑ # Awakenings)	~3yrD, intermittent D and W SS: intermittent D and W after ~3yrD

TABLE 5.1 (*continued*)

DRUG Investigators	Study Type	Subjects	Drug Regimen	Effects on Sleep Parameters			Protocol and Comments
				REMS	NREMS	Other	
COMBINATION: AMOBARBITAL + SECOBARBITAL (TUINAL®) (cont.) Kales et al, 1974	P	N = 2 Pt, insomniacs N = 10 Pt, insomniac controls	100–150 mg amobarbital + 100–150 mg secobarbital/da	↓ REMS	↓2 ↓ SWS		1 + yrD SS: 2–3 consecutive nt after 1 + yrD Comparison: 2 Pt vs 10 Pt controls
Davison et al, 1970	DE	N = 14 Hy, 8 m, 6 f, 17–37 yr	100 mg amobarbital + 100 mg secobarbital, *po* 11 PM	↓ REMS	↑1		1H,1B,1D$_1$,1D$_2$ SS: weekly D$_{1\ and\ 2}$: diphenhydramine + methaqualone, amobarbital + secobarbital DI: 1 wk
COMBINATION: NEAL-BARBITAL + SECOBARBITAL (DORMIN®) Edsjö & Dureman, 1968	DE*	N = 12 Hy	100 mg nealbarbital + 100 mg secobarbital		↓0 ↓1 ↑2	↓ S lat. ↓ Stage shifts	Protocol? (double-blind, random sequence of D) SS: 3+ nt 3 other D: secobarbital . . . DI: 3+ da English summary
Bohlin et al, 1970	DE	N = 12 Pt, anxious N = 6 Hy	100 mg nealbarbital + 100 mg secobarbital 45 min *a hs*		Pt & Hy: ↓1 ↑2 Pt: ↑4	Pt: ↑ S time ↓ S lat. ↔ Stage shifts ↓ M	Protocol? 1 other D: nitrazepam DI: 2+ da English summary

83

TABLE 5.1 (continued)

DRUG Investigators	Study Type	Subjects	Drug Regimen	Effects on Sleep Parameters			Protocol and Comments
				REMS	NREMS	Other	
BROMAZEPAM Gaillard et al., 1973	ST	N = 4 Hy m	9 mg ⎫ 27 mg ⎭	↓ REMS	↔ 2 ↓ SWS	↓ M ↑ Fast act.	1H 2BP 1D(9 mg) 1D(27 mg) 1R SS: consecutive 2 other D, same protocol: fluni-trazepam, nitrazepam DI: 3 wk
Fujii, 1973	ST	N = 4 Hy m	5 mg 1 hr a hs	↓ REMS	↔ 2 ↓ SWS	↓ S lat.	3BP 3D 2RP SS: consecutive 6 other D, same protocol: amobarbital . . . DI: ≥10 da English summary
CHLORDIAZEPOXIDE Hartmann, 1968	DE*	N = 8 Hy	100 mg 30 min a hs			↑ S time	2H ≥4B (1D₁,1D₂,1D₃,1D₄, 1D₄,1P, in random order) SS: weekly D₁₋₄: pentobarbital . . . DI: 1 wk
Perkins & Hinton, 1974	DE	N = 12 Pt, neurotic insomniacs 2 m, 10 f, 20–60 yr	20 mg 11 PM 30 mg 11 PM 40 mg 11 PM		20, 30, and 40 mg: ↑ 1 40 mg: ↑ 2 ↓ 4	20 & 40 mg: ↑ S time	2HD₁ [2D₂(different doses) 3D₃ (different doses) 1P, in Latin square design] SS: consecutive D₁₋₃: amobarbital . . . DI: 1 da
Kales & Scharf, 1973	ST	N = 4	50 mg				3BP 3D 2RP SS: consecutive

84

TABLE 5.1 (continued)

DRUG Investigators	Study Type	Subjects	Drug Regimen	Effects on Sleep Parameters			Protocol and Comments
				REMS	NREMS	Other	
CHLORDIAZEPOXIDE (cont.) Hartmann & Cravens, 1973 Cf. Cravens et al, 1974 Hartmann & Cravens, 1973	C*	N = 8 Hy m	50 mg 20 min a hs	↓ REMS ↑ REMS lat.	↑2 ↓4 ↑ Spindle den. ↑ # Spindles	↓ Stage shifts ↓ M	28D 32W SS: consecutive D1–D5, then weekly; consecutive W1–W6, then weekly P and 4 other D, same protocol: chloral hydrate, amitriptyline, chlorpromazine, reserpine DI: 32+ da
CLORAZEPATE DIPOTASSIUM Itil et al, 1972 Cf. Itil et al, 1974	DE	N = 11 Hy, slightly anxious 21–36 yr	7.5 mg tid		↑1 ↑2	↓ S lat. ↑ Fast act. ↓ Slow act.	3H ($1D_1$ $1D_2$ 1P, double-blind, in random order) SS: ? Other D: diazepam DI: ?
Karacan et al, 1973	ST*	N = 12 Hy m, 20–25 yr	7.5 mg tid	↓ REMS (R↑) → # REMS per. (R↑) (R↓ REMS lat.)	→0 ↑2 (R↓) ↓4		1H 3B 3BP 8D 3RP SS: consecutive
DIAZEPAM Saletu & Itil, 1973	P	N = 1 Pt, enuretic sleepwalker f, 52 yr	10 mg hs	↓ REM act.	↓0 → SWS		2H $1B,1D_1,1D_2,1D_3,1D_4$ SS: all H, B, and D nt D_{1-4}: diazepam, flurazepam, phenobarbital, diphenylhydantoin DI: 4 da

TABLE 5.1 (*continued*)

DRUG Investigators	Study Type	Subjects	Drug Regimen	Effects on Sleep Parameters			Protocol and Comments
				REMS	NREMS	Other	
DIAZEPAM (cont.) Itil et al, 1972	DE?	N = 11 Hy, slightly anxious 21–36 yr	5 mg tid	↑ # REMS cycles	↑ 1 ↑ 2 ↓ SWS	↓ S lat. ↑ Fast act. ↓ Slow act.	3H (1D₁ 1D₂ 1P, double-blind in random order) SS: ? Other D: clorazepate dipotassium DI: ?
Kales & Scharf, 1973	ST	N = 3 Hy	10 mg		↓ 4		3BP 3D 3RP SS: consecutive
Kales & Scharf, 1973	ST	N = 4 Pt, anxious and depressed insomniacs	5 mg 2–3 × during daytime + 5 mg hs		↓ 4	↓ S lat. ↑ # Awakenings	3BP 7D 2RP SS: consecutive nt 1–5 and 8–12
Borenstein & Cujo, 1974	ST	N = 3 Pt, insomniacs N = 3, good sleepers	10 mg im or po a hs			↑ S time ↓ # Awakenings	3+H 4B 1D 8R SS: 4B, 1D, R3, R8 3 other D, same protocol: pentobarbital. . . . DI: ?
Borenstein & Cujo, 1974	ST	N = 3 Pt, insomniacs N = 3, good sleepers	10 mg im or po a hs			↑ S time ↓ # Awakenings	3+H 4B 8D 8R SS: 4B, D3, D8, R3, R8 3 other D, same protocol: pentobarbital. . . . DI: ?
Kales & Scharf, 1973	C	N = 4 Pt, enuretic children	2.5 mg increased weekly until clinical effect ≤20 mg hs		↓ 4		4P 27D 5W SS: 3 consecutive nt intermittently

TABLE 5.1 (continued)

DRUG Investigators	Study Type	Subjects	Drug Regimen	Effects on Sleep Parameters REMS	NREMS	Other	Protocol and Comments
FLUNITRAZEPAM Gaillard et al., 1973	ST	N = 4 Hy m	2 mg 6 mg	↓ REMS ↑ REMS lat. ↑ REMS cycle ↓ REM den.	↑ 2 ↓ SWS	↓ M	1H 2BP 1D(2 mg) 1D(6 mg) 1R SS: consecutive 2 other D, same protocol: bromazepam . . . DI: 3 wk
Kales & Scharf 1973	ST	N = 4 Pt, insomniacs	2 mg *hs*	↓ REMS	↓ 0 ↓ 4	↓ S lat. ↓ # Awakenings	4BP 3D 3R SS: consecutive
Kales & Scharf, 1973	ST	N = 4 Pt, insomniacs	1 mg *hs*	↑ REMS	↓ 0	↓ # Awakenings	4BP 3D 3R SS: consecutive
Kales & Scharf 1973	ST	N = 4 Pt, insomniacs	0.25 mg *hs*		↓ SWS	↓ S lat.	4BP 7D 3R SS: consecutive
Cerone et al., 1974	ST (*2 mg)	N = 6 Pt, insomniacs m, mean 42.5 yr N = 6 Hy m, mean 26.1 yr	2 mg *hs* 4 mg *hs* (N = 3 Pt)	Hy: ↑ REMS lat.		↓ S time ↓ S lat. ↓ # Awakenings ↑ Fast act.	1H 2BP 3D(2 mg) 3P 1D(4 mg) 1P SS: consecutive
Monti et al, 1974	ST	N = 12 Pt, neurotic (9) or psychotic (3) insomniacs 6 m, 6 f, 25–62 yr	2 mg 30 min *a hs* (N = 3) 3 mg 30 min *a hs* (N = 4) 4 mg 30 min *a hs* (N = 3)	↓ REMS ↓ REMS lat.	↓ 0 ↓ SWS	↔ S time ↓ S lat. ↑ Fast act.	1H 3P 16D 2W SS: intermittent, 6D D washout 7 da prestudy

TABLE 5.1 (continued)

DRUG Investigators	Study Type	Subjects	Drug Regimen	Effects on Sleep Parameters			Protocol and Comments
				REMS	NREMS	Other	
FLURAZEPAM Rubin et al., 1973	P	N = 2 23 and 52 yr	30 mg hs		↓ 4	Normal GH peaks	2H 2B 2–3wkD 2wkW SS: 2B, D1, D2, 2 nt after 2 wk D; N = 1–1 nt after 3 wk D, 2 nt after 2 wk W GH sampled on same schedule as S
Saletu & Itil, 1973	P	N = 1 Pt, enuretic sleepwalker f, 52 yr	30 mg hs	↑ # REMS cycles	↓ 0 ↓ 3 ↓ 4	↓S lat.	2H 1B.1D$_1$,1D$_2$,1D$_3$,1D$_4$ SS: all H, B and D nt. D$_{1-4}$: diazepam, flurazepam, phenobarbital, diphenylhydantoin DI: 4 da
Hartmann, 1968	DE°	N = 10 Hy	30 mg 30 min a hs		↓ 4	↑ S time	2H ≥4B (1D$_1$,1D$_2$,1D$_3$,1D$_4$ 1D$_4$,1P, in random order) SS: weekly D$_{1-4}$: pentobarbital . . . DI: 1 wk
Itil et al., 1972	DE°	N = 10 Hy 6 m, 4 f, 20–43 yr	30 mg	↓ REMS per. length ↓ # REM bursts	↓ 0 ↓ 4	↑ Fast act. during REMS	1H 2BP [1D$_1$,1D$_2$(0.5 mg).1D$_2$(1.0 mg).1D$_2$(2.0 mg).1P, in random order] SS: every 3+ da D$_{1\ and\ 2}$: flurazepam, triazolobenzodiazepine derivative DI: 3+ da
Itil et al., 1974	ST	N = 12 Hy m	30 mg			↑ Fast act. during REMS ↑ Awakening threshold	1H 2BP (1D$_1$,1D$_2$,1D$_3$,1D$_3$,1P, in random order) SS: every 3+ da D$_{1-3}$: flurazepam, methaqualone, triazolam

TABLE 5.1 (*continued*)

DRUG Investigators	Study Type	Subjects	Drug Regimen	Effects on Sleep Parameters			Protocol and Comments
				REMS	NREMS	Other	
FLURAZEPAM (cont.)							
Kales et al, 1969	ST	N = 8	60 mg				1BP 1D 1RP SS: consecutive
Kales et al, 1970	ST	N = 4 Hy	30 mg		↓4		2H 1B 3D 2R SS: consecutive
Kales et al, 1970	ST	N = ?	60 mg	↓ REMS	↑2		1BP 1D 1RP SS: consecutive
Kales et al, 1970	ST	N = 3(?) Pt, insomniacs	30 mg		↓0 ↓4	↓ S lat.	1H 3B 14D 4W SS: consecutive nt 1–7 and 16–22
Kales et al, 1971 Cf. Allen et al., 1972	ST*	N = 8 Pt, insomniacs given D N = 4 Pt, insomniacs given P	30 mg	↓ REM den.	↓0 ↓4	↓ S lat. ↑ # Awakenings	D Pt: 4B 5D 5P 3R (N = 4) or 4B 5P 5D 3R (N = 4) P Pt: 4B 5P 5P 3R SS: consecutive
Vogel et al, 1972	ST	N = 5 Pt, insomniacs N = 5 Hy, good sleepers	15 mg (Hy) 30 mg (Pt)		Hy: ↓ SWS	Pt: ↑ S time ↓ S lat.	4BP 7D 3RP SS: consecutive Abstract
Dement et al, 1973	ST	N = 8 Pt, insomniacs given D N = 2 Pt, insomniacs given P	15 mg (N = 4) 30 mg (N = 4)	↓ REMS	↓ SWS	↑ S time ↓ S lat. 15 mg: ↓ # Awakenings	1HP 3BP 7D or 7P 3RP SS: consecutive nt 1–7 and 9–14

Table 5.1 (*continued*)

DRUG Investigators	Study Type	Subjects	Drug Regimen	Effects on Sleep Parameters REMS	NREMS	Other	Protocol and Comments
FLURAZEPAM (cont.) Fujii, 1973	ST	N = 4 Hy m	30 mg 1 hr *a hs*	↑ REMS	↑ 2, ↓ 3 + 4	↓ S lat.	3BP 3D 2RP SS: consecutive 6 other D, same protocol: amobarbital . . . DI: ≥10 da English summary
Kales & Scharf, 1973	ST	N = 4 Pt, insomniacs	15 mg	↑ REMS	↓ 0, ↓ 4	↓ S lat., ↓ # Awakenings	4BP 3D SS: consecutive
Johns & Masterton, 1974	ST°	N = 6 Hy m	15 mg		↑ 2	↑ S time, ↓ # Awakenings	1H 1BP 1D 1RP SS: consecutive
Johnson, 1975	ST	N = 5 Pt, insomniacs 1 m, 4 f, 23–42 yr	30 mg	↓ REMS, ↑ REMS lat.	↑ Spindling	↓ SW act. during 2, ↓ K-complexes during 2	4BP 7D 3RP SS: consecutive, 2BP, 3D; D7 and RP3
Kales et al., 1975	C	N = 4 Pt, insomniacs	30 mg		↓ 0, ↓ 1, ↑ 2, ↓ SWS	→ # Awakenings	Abstract
LORAZEPAM Globus et al., 1972	ST	N = 9 Hy	1–4 mg	↓ REMS	↓ 0	↓ PIP	2BP 3–4D 2R SS: ?
Borenstein & Cujo, 1974	ST	N = 3 Pt, insomniacs N = 3, good sleepers	2 mg *a hs*	↓ REMS lat.	↓ 0 (R ↑)		3+H 4B 1D 8R SS: 4B, 1D, R3, R8 3 other D, same protocol: pentobarbital . . . DI: ?

90

TABLE 5.1 (continued)

DRUG Investigators	Study Type	Subjects	Drug Regimen	Effects on Sleep Parameters			Protocol and Comments
				REMS	NREMS	Other	
LORAZEPAM (cont.) Borenstein & Cujo, 1974	ST	N = 3 Pt, insomniacs N = 3, good sleepers	2 mg a hs	↓ REMS (R ↑) ↑ REMS lat.	↓ 0 ↑ Light S ↓ Deep S	↑ S time	3+H 4B 8D 8R SS: 4B, D3, D8, R3, R8 3 other D, same protocol: pentobarbital . . . DI: ?
Globus et al., 1974	ST	N = 6 Pt, anxious insomniacs 4 m, 2 f N = 4 Hy, Pt spouses f	1–5 mg AM and 30 min a hs (Pt) 1–5 mg 30 min a hs (Hy)		↓1	↑ S time Pt: (R ↓ S time)	2H 10BP 14D 10R SS: intermittent
NITRAZEPAM Oswald & Priest, 1965	P	N = 2 Hy	15 mg	↓ REMS (R ↑)		(R ↑ S lat.)	5B 14D 80R SS: intermittent
Haider & Oswald, 1970	P	N = 2	Overdoses, ≤200 mg	↑ REMS		↑ Shifts to 0 or 1 Fast act. at 9–11 da	W SS: ?
Lehmann & Ban, 1968	DE*	N = 10 Hy 4 m, 6 f, 19–25 yr	10 mg	↓ REMS ↑ REMS lat.			1B.(1D$_1$,1D$_2$,1D$_3$,1D$_4$,1P, in Latin square design) SS: weekly D$_{1-4}$:secobarbital . . . DI: 1 wk
Haider, 1969	DE	N = 6 Hy m	10 mg	↓ REMS	↓1 ↑2 ↓SWS	↓ M	1H.1BP.1D.1R SS: weekly

TABLE 5.1 (continued)

DRUG Investigators	Study Type	Subjects	Drug Regimen	REMS	NREMS	Other	Protocol and Comments
NITRAZEPAM (cont.) Bohlin et al., 1970	DE	N = 12 Pt, anxious, N = 6 Hy	5 mg 45 min a hs		Hy: ↓1; Pt: ↓1 ↑2 ↓SWS	Pt: ↑ S time; ↑ Stage shifts; ↓ M	Protocol? 1 other D: combination—nealbarbital + secobarbital; DI: 2+ da; English summary
Allnutt & O'Connor, 1971	DE°	N = 8 Hy	5 mg		↑2		1B.1D₁,1P.1D₂,1P.1D₂,1B.1D₁, double-blind, balanced design, no consecutive active D; SS: every other nt; Other D: secobarbital; DI: 4 da
Haider & Oswald, 1971	DE°	N = 6 Hy m	10 mg	↓ REMS ↑ REMS lat.	↓1 ↑2 (SWS)	↓ S lat.; ↑ Shifts to 0; ↓ M; ↑ Fast act.; ↓ EDA	1H.(1D.1D.1P.1P, in balanced order); SS: weekly
Lechner, 1965	ST	N = 9 Hy m, 19–23 yr	10 mg		↓0 ↑2 ↓SWS	↓ S lat.	1B 1D; SS: consecutive
Gestaut et al., 1967	ST	N = 11	10 mg	↑ REMS lat.		↓ S lat.	1BP 1D; SS: ?; Abstract
Fujii, 1973 Cf. Okuma et al., 1975	ST	N = 4 Hy m	5 mg 1 hr a hs	↓ REMS (R ↑); ↓ REM den. (R ↑)	↑2 ↓3 + 4		3BP 3D 2RP; SS: consecutive; 6 other D, same protocol: amobarbital . . . ; DI: ≥10 da; English summary

$$\text{Effects on Sleep Parameters}$$

TABLE 5.1 (*continued*)

DRUG Investigators	Study Type	Subjects	Drug Regimen	Effects on Sleep Parameters			Protocol and Comments
				REMS	NREMS	Other	
NITRAZEPAM (cont.) Gaillard et al., 1973	ST	N = 4 Hy m	10 mg 30 mg	10 mg: NSC 30 mg: ↓ REMS ↑ REMS lat.	10 mg: NSC 30 mg: ↓ 2 ↓ SWS	10 mg: NSC 30 mg: ↓ M	1H 2BP 1D(10 mg) 1D(30 mg) 1R SS: consecutive 2 other D, same protocol: bromazepam . . . DI: 3 wk
Borenstein & Cujo, 1974	ST	N = 3 Pt, insomniacs N = 3, good sleepers	5 mg *a hs*	↓ REMS ↑ REMS lat.	↓ 0 ↑ 1 + 2		3+H 4B 1D 8R SS: 4B, 1D, R3, R8 3 other D, same protocol: pentobarbital . . . DI: ?
Borenstein & Cujo, 1974	ST	N = 3 Pt, insomniacs N = 3, good sleepers	5 mg *a hs*	↓ REMS ↑ REMS lat.	↓ 0 ↑ 1 + 2 ↓→ 3 + 4	S time ←→ # Awakenings ↓→	3+H 4B, 8D 8R SS: 4B, D3, D8, R3, R8 3 other D, same protocol: pentobarbital . . . DI: ?
Firth, 1974	ST	N = 4 Hy m	10 mg 20 mg	↓ REMS			2H 7BP 7D(10 mg) 7D(20 mg) 1R SS: weekly Ss awakened weekly during 2nd and 4th REMS per. for dream reports
Hata, 1975	ST	N = 4 Hy	5 mg	↓ REMS ↓ REM den.			3B 3D 2RP SS: consecutive 3 other D, same protocol: amobarbital . . . DI: ≥10 da Only REMS parameters reported English summary

TABLE 5.1 (continued)

DRUG Investigators	Study Type	Subjects	Drug Regimen	Effects on Sleep Parameters REMS	NREMS	Other	Protocol and Comments
OXAZEPAM Ehrenstein et al., 1972 Cf. Schaffler et al., 1971	DE	N = 8 Hy, nurse shift workers	10 mg	↑ REMS	↑ 1 ↑ 2 ↑ 3 ↑ 4	↑ S time	4Bnt 3Bda 3Dda SS: weekly D da S approximated B nt S Da vs nt S: ↓ S time, ↓ all stages except 0
Gaillard & Aubert, 1975	ST	N = 4 Hy	0.77 mg/kg bw 20 min *a hs* 2.31 mg/kg bw 20 min *a hs*	↓ REMS → REM act.	High D: ↑ 2	↓ K-complexes in 2 ↑ Spindle burst act. in 2	1D(low) 1D(high) 1R SS: consecutive 2 other D (pentobarbital, thioridazine), same protocol, except 1H and 2BP preceded thioridazine DI: 4 wk
TEMAZEPAM Maggini et al., 1969	ST*	N = 8 Pt, insomniac neurotics or endogenously depressed m	300 mg } 600 mg	↑ REMS	↑ 0 → 1 → 2 ↑ 3	↑ S time → S lat.	1H 1B 4D(300 mg) 4D(600 mg) SS: consecutive H and B, D4(300 mg), D4(600 mg)
TRIAZOLAM Itil et al., 1974	DE*	N = 12 Hy m	0.10 mg 0.50 mg 1.00 mg	↓ REMS ↓ Single REM act. ↓ REM bursts	↓ 4	↑ Fast act. ↓ Slow act.	1H 2BP ($1D_1,1D_2,1D_3,1D_3,1P$, in random order) SS: every 3+ da D_{1-3}: flurazepam, methaqualone, triazolam DI: 3+ da
Roth et al., 1974	ST	N = 12 Hy 25–35 yr	0.25 mg (N = 3) 0.50 mg (N = 6) } 1.00 mg (N = 3)	↑ REMS lat.	↑ 2 → 3 ↓ 4	↑ S time → S lat.	2H 2B 3D 2R SS: consecutive

94

TABLE 5.1 (continued)

DRUG Investigators	Study Type	Subjects	Drug Regimen	Effects on Sleep Parameters REMS	NREMS	Other	Protocol and Comments
TRIAZOLAM (cont.) Vogel et al., 1975	ST (°0.50 mg)	N = 9 Pt, insomniacs 6 m, 3 f, 29–54 yr	0.25 mg 30 min a hs (N = 3) 0.50 mg 30 min a hs (N = 6) 1.00 mg 30 min a hs (N = 3)	0.50 mg: ↓ REMS	0.50 mg: ↓ 0	0.50 mg: ↑ S time ↓ S lat.	4BP 7D 3R, double-blind SS: consecutive Statistical analysis for 0.50 mg dose only
Kripke & Grant, 1974	?	N = 12 Pt, insomniacs	0.60 mg			↑ S time ↓ S lat.	D P, double-blind, in random order SS: consecutive Abstract
TRIAZOLOBENZODIAZE-PINE DERIVATIVE Itil et al., 1972	DE°	N = 10 Hy 6 m, 4 f, 20–43 yr	0.50 mg 1.00 mg 2.00 mg	↓ REMS	↑ Light S	↑ Fast act. ↓ Slow act.	1H 2BP [1D₁,1D₂(0.5 mg). 1D₂(1.0 mg). 1D₂(2.0 mg).1P, in random order] SS: every 3+ da D₁ and 2: flutazepam, triazolo-benzodiazepine derivative DI: 3+ da
ALPHA CHLORALOSE Lester & Guerrero-Figueroa, 1966	DE°	N = 6 Hy	500 mg	↓ REMS ↑ REMS lat.	↑ 4	↑ Fast act.	1H.1B.1B.1D₁(120 mg).1D₁(240 mg). 1D₂,1D₃,1D₄,1B SS: weekly D₁₋₄: phenobarbital, alpha chlor-alose, thiopental, chlorpromazine DI: 1 wk
Williams et al., 1969	ST°	N = 10 Hy m	500 mg	↓ REMS (R ↑) ↑ REMS lat.	↑ SWS (R ↓) (R ↑ 1)	↓ # Awakenings (R ↑)	3B.1D 1R.1R SS: weekly, except R1 consecutive with D

95

TABLE 5.1 (*continued*)

DRUG Investigators	Study Type	Subjects	Drug Regimen	Effects on Sleep Parameters			Protocol and Comments
				REMS	N REMS	Other	
BENZAMIDE COMPOUND (SU-21707) Mendels & Chernik, 1972	ST	N = 12 Hy	350 mg (N = 6) ⎱ 700 mg (N = 6) ⎰	NSC	NSC	NSC	3P 3D 2R SS: consecutive
BENZOCTAMINE Ogunremi et al., 1973	C	N = 8 Hy m	2.5 mg tid, 20 mg hs 5.0 mg tid, 40 mg hs	(W ↑ REMS)	(W ↓ 3) (W ↓ 4)	↓ Shifts to 0 or 1 ↑ Fast act.	3wkBP 1wkD(low) 4wkD (high) 3wkWP SS: intermittent, 1BP, 1D(low), D1–D7(high), D21–D28(high), WP1–WP4, WP14–WP21 1 other D, same protocol: amobarbital Blood samples for GH and corti- costeroid levels taken via cathe- ter on nt other than S data nt
CHLORAL HYDRATE Lehmann & Ban, 1968	DE°	N = 10 Hy 4 m, 6 f, 19–25 yr	650 mg	NSC	NSC	NSC	1B.(1D$_1$,1D$_2$,1D$_3$,1D$_4$.1P, in Latin square design) SS: weekly D$_{1-4}$: secobarbital · · ·
Evans & Ogunremi, 1970	ST	N = 4 Hy m, 21–26 yr	800 mg	↓ REMS	↑ 1 ↑ 2		1H 6–13BP 7–13D 13R SS: intermittent
Kales et al, 1970	ST°	N = 10 Hy m, 20–30 yr	500 mg hs	NSC	NSC	NSC	2HP 1BP 3D 2RP SS: consecutive
Kales et al., 1970	ST°	N = 5 Hy m, 20–30 yr	1000 mg hs	NSC	NSC	NSC	2HP 1BP 3D 2RP SS: consecutive
Jovanović, 1974	ST	N = 10 Hy	1500 mg	NSC	NSC	NSC	2B 3D 3R SS: ?

96

TABLE 5.1 (continued)

DRUG Investigators	Study Type	Subjects	Drug Regimen	Effects on Sleep Parameters			Protocol and Comments
				REMS	NREMS	Other	
CHLORAL HYDRATE (cont.) Kales et al., 1970	C	N = 4 Pt, insomniacs	1000 mg			↓ S lat.	4BP 14D 4RP / SS: consecutive 4BP and D1–D3, D12–D14 and 4RP / 1 other D, same protocol: glutethimide / DI: 4 wk
Hartmann & Cravens, 1973 Cf. Hartmann & Cravens, 1973	C*	N = 8 Hy m	500 mg 20 min a hs		↓ 0	↑ S time ↓ S lat. (W ↑ M)	28D 32W / SS: consecutive D1–D5, then weekly; consecutive W1–W6, then weekly / P and 4 other D, same protocol: chlordiazepoxide . . . / DI: 32+ da
CHLORMETHIAZOLE Maxion & Schneider, 1970	DE	N = 12 Pt, chronic alcoholics post-delirium m	2.25 gm	↓ REMS ↓ REM den.	↑ NREMS		1D 1B, in balanced order / SS: consecutive
DIPHENHYDRAMINE Kales et al., 1969	ST	N = 2 Hy	50 mg	↓ REMS (R ↑)			2HP 1BP 3D 2RP / SS: consecutive
Kales et al., 1969	ST	N = 4 Hy	100 mg	↓ REMS			1BP 1D 1RP / SS: consecutive
Kales et al., 1969	ST	N = 2 Hy	50 mg	↓ REMS (R ↑)	↑ 4		2HP 1BP 3D 2RP / SS: consecutive

TABLE 5.1 (continued)

DRUG Investigators	Study Type	Subjects	Drug Regimen	Effects on Sleep Parameters			Protocol and Comments
				REMS	NREMS	Other	
GLUTETHIMIDE Williams & Agnew, 1969	DE	N = 9 Hy m	500 mg 15 min a hs	↓ REMS	↑2		1P.1D₁.1D₂, in random order; SS: all D and P; Other D: methaqualone; DI: 2 da
Allen et al., 1968	ST	N = 5 Hy 3 m, 2 f	500 mg a hs				2HP 1BP 3D 2RP; SS: consecutive; Analysis of REM den. only
Allen et al., 1968	ST	N = 4 Hy m	1000 mg a hs	↓ REM den.			1BP 1D 1RP; SS: consecutive; Analysis of REM den. only
Rubin et al., 1969	ST	N = 4 Hy	1000 mg	↓ REMS (R↑); ↓ REM den.		↓ 17-hydroxy-corticosteroids	1BP 1D 1RP; SS: consecutive
Goldstein et al., 1970 Cf. Goldstein et al., 1971	ST*	N = 10 Pt, insomniacs m, 21–54 yr	500 mg	↓ REMS (R↑); ↑ REMS lat.	→0 ↑2	(R↑ # Awakenings)	2H 1B 3D 4RP; SS: consecutive; 1 other D, same protocol, in balanced order: methaqualone; DI: 3–8 wk
Kales et al., 1970	ST	N = 5 Hy m, 21–30 yr	500 mg	↓ REMS (R↑); ↑ REMS lat.; ↑ REM bursts	←2 →4		2HP 1BP 3D 2RP; SS: consecutive
Kales et al., 1969	ST	N = 4 Hy m, 21–30 yr	1000 mg	↓ REMS (R↑); ↑ REMS lat.; ↓ # REMS per.			1BP 1D 1RP; SS: consecutive
Kales et al., 1970	C	N = 4 Pt, insomniacs	500 mg	↓ REMS (R↑)			4BP 14D 4RP; SS: consecutive 4BP and D1–D3, D12–D14 and 4RP; 1 other D, same protocol: chloral hydrate; DI: 4 wk

98

TABLE 5.1 (*continued*)

DRUG Investigators	Study Type	Subjects	Drug Regimen	Effects on Sleep Parameters			Protocol and Comments
				REMS	NREMS	Other	
GLUTETHIMIDE (cont.) Kales et al., 1974	C	N = 3 Pt, insomniacs on D N = 10 Pt, insomniac controls 34–40 yr	500–1000 mg/nt	↓ REMS			1 yr D SS: 2–3 nt after 1 yr D Comparison: Pt on D vs Pt controls
HEXAPROPYMATE Risberg et al., 1972	DE*	N = 16 Hy 8 m, 8 f, 20–30 yr	400 mg	↓ REMS ↑ REMS lat.	↓ 0 ↑ 2	↑ S time ↓ S lat.	(1H 2D),(1H 2P), in balanced order SS: consecutive, 1 wk between D and P
MEBUTAMATE Whitsett et al., 1974	ST*	N = 10 Hy, inmates m, 24–39 yr	600 mg hs	↓ REMS ↑ REMS lat. ↑ # REMS per. ↓ REM den.	↑ 2 ↑ 4	↑ Fast act.	2H 2B 3D 2R SS: consecutive
MEPROBAMATE Freemon et al., 1965	DE*	N = 8 Hy	400 mg 9 PM, 800 mg hs	↓ REMS	↓ 1 ↑ 2		1H,1D,1P, double-blind SS: all nt (4–7 da between)
Williams & Agnew, 1969	DE	N = 27 Hy m	400 mg 15 min a hs (N = 18) 800 mg 15 min a hs (N = 9)	NSC	NSC	NSC	1P,1D₁,1D₂, in random order SS: all D and P Other D: pentobarbital DI: 2 da 2 studies of 400 mg (N = 9 for each) and 1 study of 800 mg, all with same protocol

99

TABLE 5.1 (continued)

DRUG / Investigators	Study Type	Subjects	Drug Regimen	Effects on Sleep Parameters			Protocol and Comments
				REMS	NREMS	Other	
METHAQUALONE Williams & Agnew, 1969	DE	N = 9 Hy m	300 mg 15 min *a hs*	NSC	NSC	NSC	1P.1D$_1$.1D$_2$, in random order SS: all D and P Other D: glutethimide DI: 2 da
Itil et al., 1974	DE°	N = 12 Hy m	300 mg	↓ REM bursts	↑ 1 ↑ 2 ↓ 4	↑ Fast act. ↓ Slow act.	1H 2BP (1D$_1$,1D$_2$,1D$_3$,1D$_3$,1P, in random order) SS: every 3+ da D$_{1-3}$: flurazepam . . . DI: 3+ da
Risberg et al., 1975	DE°	N = 6 Hy m	250 mg	↓ REMS ↓ REM den.	↑ 2		2H.1D.1P SS: weekly
Goldstein et al., 1970 Cf. Goldstein et al., 1971	ST°	N = 10 Pt, insomniacs m, 21–54 yr	300 mg	(R ↑ REMS)	↓ 0 ↑ 2 ↓ 4	↓ S lat.	2H 1B 3D 4RP SS: consecutive 1 other D, same protocol, in balanced order: glutethimide DI: 3–8 wk
Kales et al., 1970	ST°	N = 5 Hy m, 20–30 yr	150 mg	NSC	NSC	NSC	2HP 1BP 3D 2RP SS: consecutive
Kales et al., 1970	ST°	N = 5 Hy m, 20–30 yr	300 mg	↓ REMS (R ↑)			2HP 1BP 3D 2RP SS: consecutive
Rechtschaffen et al., 1970	ST	N = 6 Hy m	150 mg 45 min *a hs*	↑ REM den.			2BP 3D 2R SS: consecutive Abstract
Risberg et al., 1975	ST	N = 4 Hy m	250 mg	NSC	NSC	NSC	2H 2BP 3D 3R SS: consecutive
METHYPRYLON Kales et al., 1970	ST°	N = 7 Hy m, 21–30 yr	300 mg	↓ REMS (R ↑)			2HP 1BP 3D 2RP SS: consecutive

TABLE 5.1 (continued)

DRUG Investigators	Study Type	Subjects	Drug Regimen	REMS	NREMS	Other	Protocol and Comments
				Effects on Sleep Parameters			
PERLAPINE Allen & Oswald, 1973	P	N = 2 Hy m	10 mg			↓ Shifts to 0 or 1	2HP 4BP 1wkD 1wkRP SS: intermittent B; D1, D2, D4; 3RP
Williams et al., 1974	ST	N = 12	20 mg 30 min *a hs*	↑ REMS lat.		↓ S lat. ↓ # Awakenings ↓ Stage shifts	1H 3B 3BP 9D 3RP SS: consecutive Abstract
Allen & Oswald, 1973	C	N = 5 Hy m	10 mg (N = 3) ⎱ 20 mg (N = 2) ⎰	↓ REMS (W ↑)	↓ 0	↓ Shifts to 0 or 1	1wkB 3wkD 2wkW SS: B1, B2, B3, B5, D1, D2, D3, D5, W1, W2, W3, W5
TRICLOFOS Zung, 1973	ST°	N = 5 Hy 3 m, 2 f, 20–45 yr	1000 mg *a hs*	NSC	NSC	NSC	4B.2D₁ 2RP,2D₂ SS: 2–4 consecutive nt of 3 consecutive wk D₁ ₐₙₐ ₂: phenobarbital, triclofos DI: 6 da
COMBINATION: DIPHEN-HYDRAMINE + METHAQUALONE (MANDRAX®) Davison et al., 1970	DE	N = 14 Hy 8 m, 6 f, 17–37 yr	250 mg methaqualone + 25 mg diphenhydramine *po* 11 PM			↑ S time	1H.1B.1D₁.1D₂ SS: weekly D₁ ₐₙₐ ₂: diphenhydramine + methaqualone, amobarbital + secobarbital DI: 1 wk
Jovanović, 1973	ST°	N = 10 Hy	250 mg methaqualone + 25 mg diphenhydramine	↓ REMS (R ↑) ↑ REMS lat.	↓ Superficial S stages ↑ Deep S stages	↓ S lat.	3BP 4D 3RP SS: ? English summary

101

References

Allen, C.; A. Kales; and R. J. Berger. An analysis of the effect of glutethimide on REM density. *Psychonomic Science* 12 (1968): 329–30.

Allen, C.; M. B. Scharf; and A. Kales. The effect of flurazepam (Dalmane) administration and withdrawal on REM density. Abstract. *Psychophysiology* 9 (1972): 92–93.

Allen, S. R., and I. Oswald. The effects of perlapine on sleep. *Psychopharmacologia* 32 (1973): 1-9.

Allnutt, M. F., and P. J. O'Connor. Comparison of the encephalographic, behavioral and subjective correlates of natural and drug-induced sleep at atypical hours. *Aerosp. Med.* 42 (1971): 1006–10.

Baeckeland, F. Pentobarbital and dextroamphetamine sulfate: Effects on the sleep cycle in man. *Psychopharmacologia* 11 (1967): 388–96.

Bixler, E. O.; M. B. Scharf; L. A. Leo; and A. Kales. Hypnotic drugs and performance: A review of theoretical and methodical considerations. In Kagan, F.; T. Harwood; K. Rickels; A. D. Rudzik; and H. Sorer, eds. *Hypnotics: Methods of Development and Evaluation*, pp. 175–94. New York: Spectrum publications, 1975.

Bohlin, G.; G. Wikmark; and I. Dureman. Självskattade och fysiologiskt registrerade effekter av två sömnmedel (nitrazepam och dormin). *Särtryck ur Nordisk Medicin* 83 (1970): 137–42.

Borenstein, P., and P. Cujo. Influence of barbiturates and benzodiazepines on the sleep EEG. In *Psychotropic Drugs and the Human EEG. Modern Problems of Pharmacopsychiatry*, edited by T. M. Itil, 8: 182–92. Basel: Karger, 1974.

Brazier, M. A. B. Electroencephalographic studies of sleep in man. In Dillon, J. B., C. M. Ballinger, eds. *Anesthesiology and the Nervous System. Proceedings of the 1965 Western Biennial Conference on Anesthesiology*, pp. 106–28. Salt Lake City: University of Utah Press, 1966.

Brazier, M. A. B., and H. K. Beecher. Alpha content of the electroencephalogram in relation to movements made in sleep, and effect of a sedative on this type of motility. *J. Appl. Physiol.* 4 (1952): 819–25.

Cerone, G.; F. Cirignotta; G. Coccagna; F. F. Milone; P. Lion; A. Lorizio; E. Lugaresi; M. Mantovani; A. Muratorio; L. Murri; R. Mutani; and A. Riccio. All-night polygraphic recordings on the hypnotic effects of a new benzodiazepine: Flunitrazepam (RO 5–4200, Rohypnol) *Europ. Neurol.* 11 (1974): 172–79.

Cravens, J.; J. Sheehan; and E. Hartmann. The sleep spindle: Effects of chlordiazepoxide; effects of other conditions. Abstract. In Chase, M. H.; W. C. Stern; and P. L. Walter, eds., *Sleep Research*, 3: 48. Los Angeles, Brain Information Service/Brain Research Institute University of California, 1974.

Davison, K.; J. P. Duffy; and J. W. Osselton. A comparison of sleep patterns in natural and mandrax- and tuinal-induced sleep. *Can. Med. Assoc. J.* 102: 506–08, 1970.

Dement, W. C.; V. P. Zarcone; E. Hoddes; H. Smythe; and M. Carskadon. Sleep laboratory and clinical studies with flurazepam. In Garattini, S.; E. Mussini; and L. O. Randall, eds. *The Benzodiazepines*, pp. 599–611. New York: Raven Press, 1973.

Edsjö, K., and I. Dureman. Experimentalla sömnstudier med enkla och kombinerade barbitursyraderivat. *Nord. Med.* 20 (1968): 805–10.

Ehrenstein, W. von; K. Schaffler; and W. Müller-Limmroth. Die Wirkung von Oxazepam auf den gestörten Tagschlaf nach Nachtschichtarbeit. *Arzneim. Forsch.* 22 (1972): 421–27.

Evans, J. I., and S. A. Lewis. Drug withdrawal state: An EEG sleep study. *Arch. Gen. Psychiatry* 19: 631–34, 1968.

Evans, J. I.; S. A. Lewis; I. A. M. Gibb; and M. Cheetham. Sleep and barbiturates: Some experiments and observations. *Br. Med. J.* 4 (1968): 291–93.

Evans, J. I., and O. Ogunremi. Sleep and hypnotics: Further experiments. *Br. Med. J.* 3 (1970): 310–13.

Feinberg, I.; S. Hibi; C. Cavness; and J. March. Absence of REM rebound after barbiturate withdrawal. *Science* 185 (1974): 534–35.

Feinberg, I.; P. H. Wender; R. L. Koresko; F. Gottlieb; and J. A. Piehuta. Differential effects of chlorpromazine and phenobarbital on EEG sleep patterns. *J. Psychiatr. Res.* 7 (1969): 101–09.

Firth, H. Sleeping pills and dream content. *Br. J. Psychiatry* 124 (1974): 547–53.

Freemon, F. R.; H. W. Agnew, Jr.; and R. L. Williams. An electroencephalographic study of the effects of meprobamate on human sleep. *Clin. Pharmacol. Ther.* 6 (1965): 172–76.

Fujii, S. Effects of some psychotropic and hypnotic drugs on the human nocturnal sleep. *Psychiatr. Neurol. Jap.* 75 (1973): 545–73.

Gaillard, J.-M., and C. Aubert. Specificity of benzodiazepine action on human sleep confirmed. Another contribution of automatic analysis of polygraph recordings. *Biol. Psychiatry* 101 (1975): 185–97.

Gaillard, J.-M.; P. Schulz; and R. Tissot. Effects of three benziodiazepines (nitrazepam, flunitrazepam and bromazepam) on sleep of normal subjects, studies with an automatic sleep scoring system. *Pharmakopsychiatrie Neuro-Psychopharmakologie* 6 (1973): 207–17.

Gastaut, H.; H. Lob; and J. J. Papy. Action of mogadon on the stages of REM sleep. Abstract. *Electroencephalogr. Clin. Neurophysiol.* 23 (1967): 288.

Globus, G. G.; E. C. Phoebus; W. Fishbein; R. Boyd; and T. Leventhal. The effect of lorazepam on sleep. *J. Clin. Pharmacol.* 12 (1972): 331–36.

Globus, G.; E. Phoebus; J. Humphries; R. Boyd; D. Gaffney; and S. Gaffney. The effect of lorazepam on anxious insomniacs' sleep as recorded in the home environment. *J. Clin. Pharmacol.* 14 (1974): 192–201.

Goldstein, L.; J. Graedon; D. Willard; F. Goldstein; and R. R. Smith. A comparative study of the effects of methaqualone and glutethimide on sleep in male chronic insomniacs. *J. Clin. Pharmacol.* 110 (1970): 258–68.

Goldstein, L.; N. W. Stoltzfus; and R. R. Smith. An analysis of the effects of methaqualone and glutethimide on sleep in insomniac subjects. *Res. Commun. Chem. Pathol. Pharmacol.* 2 (1971): 927–33.

Haider, I. Effects of a hypnotic (sodium amylobarbitone 200 mg) on human sleep—an electroencephalographic study. *Pakistan Medical Forum* 4 no. 8 (1969): 21–30.

———. Effects of a non-barbiturate hypnotic (nitrazepam-mogadon) on human sleep—an electroencephalographic study. *Pakistan Medical Forum* 4 no. 11 (1969): 13–28.

Haider, I., and I. Oswald. Late brain recovery processes after drug overdose. *Br. Med. J.* 2 (1970): 318–22.

———. Effects of amylobarbitone and nitrazepam on the electrodermogram and other features of sleep. *Br. J. Psychiatry* 118 (1971): 519–22.

Hartmann, E. The effect of four drugs on sleep patterns in man. *Psychopharmacologia* 12 (1968): 346–53.

Hartmann, E., and J. Cravens. The effects of long-term administration of psychotropic drugs on human sleep. I. Methodology and the effects of placebo. *Psychopharmacologia* 33 (1973): 153–67.

———. The effects of long-term administration of psychotropic drugs on human sleep. II. The effects of reserpine. *Psychopharmacologia* 33 (1973): 169–84.

———. The effects of long-term administration of psychotropic drugs on human sleep. III. The effects of amitriptyline. *Psychopharmacologia* 33 (1973): 185–202.

———. The effects of long-term administration of psychotropic drugs on human sleep. IV. The effects of chlorpromazine. *Psychopharmacologia* 33 (1973): 203–18.

———. The effects of long-term administration of psychotropic drugs on human sleep. V. The effects of chloral hydrate. *Psychopharmacologia* 33 (1973): 219–32.

———. The effects of long-term administration of psychotropic drugs on human sleep. VI. The effects of chlordiazepoxide. *Psychopharmacologia* 33 (1973): 233–45.

Hata, H. Effects of some neuro-active drugs on REM sleep and rapid eye movements during REM sleep in man. *Psychiatr. Neurol. Jap.* 77 (1975): 29–52.

Itil, T. M. Effects of psychotropic drugs on computer "sleep prints" in man. In Cerletti, A., ed. *The Present Status of Psychotropic Drugs, Proceedings of the VI International Congress of the CINP, Tarragona, April 1968*, pp. 211–27. Excerpta Medica International Congress Series, no. 180. Amsterdam, Excerpta Medical Foundation, 1969.

Itil, T. M.; B. Saletu; S. Akpinar. Classification of psychotropic drugs based on digital computer sleep prints. In Itil, T. M., ed., *Psychotropic Drugs and the Human EEG. Mod. Probl. Pharmacopsychiat*, pp. 193–215. Basel: Karger, 1974.

Itil, T. M.; B. Saletu; and J. Marasa. Digital computer analyzed sleep electroencephalogram (sleep prints) in predicting anxiolytic properties of clorazepate dipotassium (tranxene). *Curr. Ther. Res.* 14 (1972): 415–27.

———. Determination of drug-induced changes in sleep quality based on digital computer "sleep prints." *Pharmakopsychiatrie Neuro-Psychopharmakologie* 7 (1974): 265–80.

Itil, T. M.; B. Saletu; J. Marasa; and A. N. Mucciardi. Digital com-

puter analyzed awake and sleep EEG (sleep prints) in predicting the effects of a triazolobenzodiazepine (U-31889). *Pharmakopsychiatrie Neuro-Psychopharmakologie* 5 (1972): 225–40.

Johns, M. W., and J. P. Masterton. Effect of flurazepam on sleep
in the laboratory. *Pharmacology* 11 (1974): 358–64.

Johnson, L. C. Effect of flurazepam on sleep spindles and K-complexes. Abstract. Second International Sleep Research Congress,
Edinburgh, Scotland, June 30–July 4, 1975.

Jovanović, U. J. Der Effekt einer Kombination von Methaqualon
und Diphenhydramin auf Schlaf gesunder Menschen. *Med.
Klin.* 68 (1973): 334–39.

———. Zum Problem der Effekte zentral-wirkender Pharmaka auf
den REM-Anteil des Schlafs. *Fortschr. Med.* 92 (1974): 1090–
94.

Kales, A.; C. Allen; M. B. Scharf; and J. D. Kales. Hypnotic drugs
and their effectiveness. III. All-night EEG studies of insomniac
subjects. *Arch. Gen. Psychiatry* 23 (1970): 226–32.

Kales, A.; E. O. Bixler; T.-L. Tan; M. B. Scharf; and J. D. Kales.
Chronic hypnotic-drug use ineffectiveness, drug-withdrawal insomnia, and dependence. *JAMA* 227 (1974): 513–17.

Kales, A.; G. Heuser; J. D. Kales; W. H. Rickles, Jr.; R. T. Rubin;
M. B. Scharf; J. T. Ungerleider; and W. D. Winters. Drug de-
pendency: Investigations of stimulants and depressants. *Ann.
Intern. Med.* 70 (1969): 591–614.

Kales, A.; J. D. Kales; E. O. Bixler; and M. D. Scharf. Effectiveness of hypnotic drugs with prolonged use: Flurazepam and
pentobarbital. *Clin. Pharmacol. Ther.* 18 (1975): 356–63.

Kales, A.; J. D. Kales; A. Jacobson; R. D. Walter; and T. E. Wilson. Effects of methyprylon and pentobarbital on sleep patterns.
Abstract. *Electroencephalogr. Clin. Neurophysio.* 24 (1968):
397.

Kales, A.; J. D. Kales; M. B. Scharf; and T.-L. Tan. Hypnotics and
altered sleep-dream patterns. II. All-night EEG studies of chloral
hydrate, flurazepam, and methaqualone. *Arch. Gen. Psychiatry*
23 (1970): 219–25.

Kales, A.; E. J. Malmstrom; W. H. Rickles; J. Henley; T.-L. Tan;
B. Stadel; and F. S. Hoedemaker. Sleep patterns of a pentobarbital addict: Before and after withdrawal. *Psychophysiology* 5
(1968): 208.

Kales, A.; E. J. Malmstrom; and T.-L. Tan. Drugs and dreaming. In Abt, E., and B. F. Riess, eds. *Progress in Clinical Psychology,* pp. 154–67. New York: Grune & Stratton, 1969.

Kales, A.; T. A. Preston; T.-L. Tan; and C. Allen. Hypnotics and altered sleep-dream patterns. I. All-night studies of glutethimide, methyprylon, and pentobarbital. *Arch. Gen. Psychiatry* 23 (1970): 211–18.

Kales, A., and M. B. Scharf. Sleep laboratory and clinical studies of the effects of benzodiazepines on sleep: Flurazepam, diazepam, chlordiazepoxide, and RO 5–4200. In Garattini, S.; E. Mussini; and L. O. Randall, eds. *The Benzodiazepines,* pp. 577–98. New York: Raven Press, 1973.

Kales, J.; A. Kales; E. O. Bixler; and E. S. Slye. Effects of placebo and flurazepam on sleep patterns in insomniac subjects. *Clin. Pharmacol. Ther.* 12 (1971): 691–97.

Karacan, I.; G. S. O'Brien; R. L. Williams; P. J. Salis, and J. I. Thornby. Methodology for electroencephalographic sleep evaluation of drugs. In Koella, W. P., and P. Levin, eds. *Sleep: Physiology, Biochemistry, Psychology, Pharmacology, Clinical Implications. Proceedings of the First European Congress on Sleep Research, Basel, October 3–6, 1972,* pp. 463-76. Basel: Karger, 1973.

Kay, D. C.; D. R. Jasinski; R. B. Eisenstein; and O. A. Kelly. Quantified human sleep after pentobarbital. *Clin. Pharmacol. Ther.* 13 (1972): 221–31.

Kripke, D. F., and I. Grant. A double-blind study of triazolam. Abstract. In Chase, M. H.; W. C. Stern; and P. L. Walter, eds. *Sleep Research,* 3: 57. Los Angeles, Brain Information Service/ Brain Research Institute, University of California, 1974.

Lechner, H. Effect of mogadon on nighttime sleep. *Prog. Brain Res.* 18 (1965): 225–26.

Lehmann, H. E., and T. A. Ban. The effect of hypnotics on rapid eye movement (REM). *Internationale Zeitschrift für klinische Pharmakologie, Therapie und Toxikologie* 1 (1968): 424–27.

Lester, B. K.; J. D. Coulter; L. C. Cowden; and H. L. Williams. Secobarbital and nocturnal physiological patterns. *Psychopharmacologia* 13 (1968): 275–86.

Lester, B. K. and R. Guerrero Figueroa. Effects of some drugs on electroencephalographic fast activity and dream time. *Psychophysiology* 2 (1966): 224–36.

The Sleeping Pill

Lester, L. A new method for the determination of the effectiveness of sleep-inducing agents in humans. *Compr. Psychiatry* 1 (1960) 301–07.

Maggini, C.; M. Murri; and G. Sacchetti. Evaluation of the effectiveness of temazepam on the insomnia of patients with neurosis and endogenous depression. *Arzneim. Forsch.* 19 (1969): 1647–52.

Maxion, H., and E. Schneider. Der EinfluB von Chlormethiazol (Distraneurin) auf das Schlaf-Electroencephalogramm nach Alkoholdelir. *Pharmakopsychiatrie Neuro-Psychopharmakologie* 3 (1970): 233–38.

Mendels, J., and D. A. Chernik. The effects of SU-21707 on the sleep electroencephalogram of normal subjects. *Curr. Ther. Res.* 14 (1972): 454–60.

Monti, J. M.; H. M. Trenchi; F. Morales; and L. Monti. Flunitrazepam and sleep cycle in insomniac patients. *Psychopharmacologia* 35 (1974): 371–79.

Ogunremi, O. O.; L. Adamson; V. Březinová; W. M. Hunter; A. W. MacLean; I. Oswald; and I. W. Percy-Robb. Two anti-anxiety drugs: A psychoneuroendocrine study. *Br. Med. J.* 2 (1973): 202–05.

Okuma, T.; N. Hata; and S. Fujii. Differential effects of chlorpromazine, imipramine, nitrazepam and amobarbital on REM sleep and REM density in man. *Folia. Psychiatr. Neurol. Jap.* 29 (1975): 25–37.

Oswald, I.; R. J. Berger; R. A. Jaramillo; K. M. G. Keddie; P. C. Olley; and G. B. Plunkett. Melancholia and barbiturates. A controlled EEG, body and eye movement study of sleep. *Br. J. Psychiatry* 109 (1963): 66–78.

Oswald, I., and R. G. Priest. Five weeks to escape the sleeping-pill habit. *Br. Med. J.* 2 (1965): 1093–99.

Perkins, R., and J. Hinton. Sedative or tranquillizer? A comparison of the hypnotic effects of chlordiazepoxide and amylobarbitone sodium. *Br. J. Psychiatry* 124 (1974): 435–39.

Rechtschaffen, A., and L. Maron. The effect of amphetamine on the sleep cycle. *Electroencephalogr. Clin. Neurophysiol.* 16 (1964): 438–45.

Rechtschaffen, A.; T. M. Robinson; and M. Z. Wincor. The effect of methaqualone on nocturnal sleep. *Psychophysiology* 7 (1970): 346.

Risberg, A.-M.; J. Risberg; D. Elmqvist; and D. H. Ingvar. Effects of dixyrazine and methaqualone on the sleep pattern in normal man. *Eur. J. Clin. Pharmacol.* 8 (1975): 227–31.

Risberg, A.-M.; J. Risberg; and D. H. Ingvar. The effects of hexapropymate upon sleep in normal man measured with a polygraphic technique. *J. Clin. Pharmacol.* 4 (1972): 241–44.

Roth, T.; M. Kramer; and J. L. Schwartz. Triazolam: A sleep laboratory study of a new benzodiazepine hypnotic. *Curr. Ther. Res.* 16 (1974): 117–23.

Rubin, R. T.; P. R. Gouin; A. T. Arenander; and R. E. Poland. Human growth hormone release during sleep following prolonged flurazepam administration. *Research Communications in Chemical Pathology and Pharmacology* 6 (1973): 331–34.

Rubin, R. T.; A. Kales; and B. R. Clark. Decreased 17-hydroxycorticosteroid and VMA excretion during sleep following glutethimide administration in man. *Life Sci.* (I) 8 (1969): 959–64.

Saletu, B., and T. M. Itil. Digital computer "sleep prints"–an indicator of the most effective drug treatment of somnambulism. *Clinical Electroencephalography* 4 (1973): 33–41.

Schaffler, K.-D.; W. Ehrenstein; W. Müller-Limmroth; and C. Thébaud. Psychopharmacological influence on day sleep after night shift. *Gegenbaurs. Morphol. Jahrb.* 117 (1971): 107–14.

Takahashi, Y.; D. M. Kipnis; and W. H. Daughaday. Growth hormone secretion during sleep. *J. Clin. Invest.* 47 (1968): 2079–90.

Vogel, G. W.; J. Hickman: A. Thurmond; B. Barrowclough; and D. Giesler. The effect of dalmane (flurazepam) on the sleep cycle of good and poor sleepers. Abstract. *Psychophysiology* 9 (1972): 96.

Vogel, G., A. Thurmond; P. Gibbons; K. Edwards; K. B. Sloan; and K. Sexton. The effect of triazolam on the sleep of insomniacs. *Psychopharmacologia* 41 (1975): 65–69.

Whitsett, T. L.; H. J. Hoyt; A. W. Czerwinski; and M. L. Clark. Effects of mebutamate on the electroencephalographic sleep profile. *Clin. Pharmacol. Ther.* 15 (1974): 51–58.

Williams, H. L.; B. K. Lester; and J. D. Coulter. Alpha chloralose and nocturnal physiological patterns. *Psychopharmacologia* 15 (1969): 28–38.

Williams, R. L. Effects of Dormison compared to seconal for sleep electroencephalograms. *Electroencephalogr. Clin. Neurophysiol.* 6 (1954): 497–98.

Williams, R. L., and H. W. Agnew, Jr. The effects of drugs on the EEG sleep patterns of normal humans. *Exp. Med. Surg.* 27 (1969): 53–64.

Williams, R. L.; H. W. Agnew, Jr.; and W. B. Webb. Effects of drugs and disease on the EEG patterns in human sleep. *Proceedings of the IV World Congress of Psychiatry, Madrid, 5–11, September 1966. Excerpta Medica International Congress Series No. 150*, pp. 3093–96. Amsterdam: Excerpta Medica Foundation, 1968.

Williams, R. L.; I. Karacan; J. I. Thornby; P. J. Salis; A. M. Anch; M. Okawa; A. B. Blackburn; and L. E. Beutler. The effect of perlapine on EEG sleep patterns of insomniacs. Abstract. In Chase, M. H.; W. C. Stern; and P. L. Walter, eds. *Sleep Research,* 3: 68. Los Angeles: Brain Information Service/Brain Research Institute, University of California, 1974.

Zung, W. W. K. The effect of placebo and drugs on human sleep. *Biol. Psychiatry* 6 (1973): 89–92.

6

Insomnia

In this chapter, I shall attempt to define *insomnia*, present a current classification of insomnia and its causes, suggest a pathophysiology of insomnia, and discuss its treatment. Along the way I shall also consider a condition sometimes called "pseudoinsomnia" and the rare condition of "total insomnia."

All this is only my own best attempt at making sense of a poorly understood problem. I am forced to use clinical experience and clinical "feel" when scientific data are lacking. For our ignorance about insomnia is immense: despite the frequency of this condition, we are only at the very beginnings of any scientific knowledge about it.

There is one major point which I hope will become obvious from the following discussion, but just in case it doesn't, I'll state it here. Insomnia is not an illness for which a sleeping pill is the cure; insomnia is a symptom (a complaint) which can have many different causes. The causes are just beginning to be investigated and understood, and new ones are being discovered every year.

DEFINITION

Insomnia refers to difficulty in sleeping. There are basically only two complaints: difficulty falling asleep and difficulty remaining asleep. Insomnia must be clearly differentiated from merely "short sleep." There is a considerable range of sleep times and sleep requirements among normal individuals who have no complaints. My laboratory, in collaboration with Frederick Baekeland's laboratory in New York, studied in detail persons who get along well on about five hours of sleep. We found certain personality types and physiological patterns in these "short sleepers"; but these people are not ill. Short sleepers should not require medical attention, although they may occasionally appear in a doctor's office if they have been convinced by someone else that their sleep durations are unnatural and must be unhealthy.

Insomnia is an extremely common condition; as we have seen, in the course of a year, up to 30 percent of the population suffers from insomnia and seeks help for it. I shall try to establish in the following discussion that, although insomnia is extremely common, no treatment may be required in many cases, and in many others a careful diagnostic work-up will reveal specific causes of the insomnia so that specific treatment aimed at the cause may be used. The prescription of a sleeping pill as a long-term remedy for insomnia should be a relatively rare occurrence.

SOME CAUSES OF INSOMNIA

Table 6.1 presents a classification or nosology of the insomnias and my best current attempt to define causative factors. The broad grouping by chief complaint is still useful: difficulty falling asleep (sleep-onset insomnia) versus difficulty remaining asleep. Some textbooks refer to three symptoms: difficulty in falling asleep, frequent awakenings during the night, and early-morning awakening. However, in my experience the second and third symptoms almost always occur together and are associated with the same probable causes. Thus I have combined them in the symptom "difficulty in remaining asleep."*

The three columns in table 6.1 represent broad categories of etiological factors. These lists are in no way final or static:

---

* Some researchers have suggested that the distinction between "difficulty falling asleep" and "difficulty remaining asleep" is simply a matter of age. Difficulty falling asleep is certainly more common in the young, while difficulty remaining asleep is more frequently seen in older people, but there are enough exceptions that I believe the distinction is worth keeping.

TABLE 6.1

Classifications of Insomnia

	Insomnias Secondary to Medical Conditions	Insomnias Secondary to Psychiatric or Environmental Conditions	Idiopathic Insomnias (Cause Unknown)
Difficulty falling asleep	Any painful or uncomfortable condition	Anxiety, simple or transient Anxiety, chronic, neurotic Anxiety, prepsychotic Tension-anxiety, muscular Environmental changes	Idiopathic sleep-onset insomnia (rare)
	Brainstem lesions (The conditions listed below will at times also produce difficulty in falling asleep.)	Conditioned (habit) insomnia	
Difficulty remaining asleep	Sleep apnea	Depression	Idiopathic difficulty in remaining asleep
	Nocturnal myoclonus	Especially endogenous or primary depression Environmental change	
	Episodic events Direct drug effects Drug withdrawal effects Endocrine abnormalities Metabolic abnormalities Brainstem or hypothalamic lesions Dietary factors Other		

growing attention to insomnia in sleep laboratory studies has gradually increased the number of conditions listed in the columns on the left—insomnias resulting from medical and psychiatric or environmental conditions. I believe that not more than 20 percent of insomniac patients now need to be classified in the righthand column as "idiopathic." Eventually, as more is learned about the biology of the brain, the first two columns will also merge and we shall be speaking simply of the pathophysiology or development of insomnia (pp. 118–20).

Many of the causes of insomnia listed in the table are fairly obvious. Any painful or uncomfortable condition can produce insomnia, usually difficulty in falling asleep, and this is very common among the insomniacs seen by a general or family practitioner. Some people are able to ignore bodily pain or discomfort during a busy day and only become aware of it when trying to get to sleep in the evening.

Sleep apnea, though infrequent, is important since it can be life-threatening and is usually treatable. This is a recently discovered condition in which the patient's respiration ceases completely a number of times during the night; he then awakens, takes a few breaths, and falls asleep again; the process repeats itself, sometimes hundreds of times per night. Sleep is obviously poor and may result in complaints of insomnia, though more frequently the complaint is excessive daytime sleepiness. Reports from a bed partner may make one suspect this diagnosis, but it must be confirmed by sleep laboratory recordings, including recordings of respiration. Sleep apnea is sometimes produced by direct physical problems in the tissues of the neck or pharynx (peripheral type) and sometimes by problems in the brainstem respiratory centers (central type).

Nocturnal myoclonus is a neuromuscular abnormality which manifests itself in sudden repeated contractions of one or more muscle groups during sleep. Most commonly there are periods of repeated jerking of the legs, but head movements are the chief symptom in some cases. Nocturnal myoclonus is a cause of insomnia when the movements repeatedly awaken the sleeper; in many cases the sleeper does not awaken, and the myoclonus is only disturbing to the bed partner.

Dietary factors as causes for insomnia may be important but have hardly yet been investigated. General malnutrition can play a role in producing insomnia, although in countries where malnutrition is a major problem its far more serious consequences, such as susceptibility to infectious illnesses, overshadow the insomnia.] One specific type of malnutrition that occurs in rural Mexicans and Latin Americans deserves further study in terms of its relationship to insomnia. The overall food intake of these groups may be adequate, but since corn is used as their total or almost total source of protein, they develop a tryptophan deficiency as corn protein is more or less adequate with respect to all amino acids except for l-tryptophan—and tryptophan deficiency can produce insomnia. In such cases, addition of l-tryptophan to the diet would help to normalize the ratio of amino acids and would be a physiological replacement therapy in the treatment of insomnia, as well as a treatment for other deficiency symptoms. Many other aspects of diet could be of importance too. For instance, there are hints from clinical experience and case reports that the body's supplies of calcium, magnesium, and other metals are important for sleep, and that alteration can produce insomnia; but this has not as yet been adequately studied.

Several of the "psychiatric" causes of insomnia are especially frequent. In a young, medically healthy person, some form of anxiety is the chief cause of insomnia. It is worth exploring the source of anxiety in detail since treatment will be directly affected by what it is. It can sometimes be simple conscious worry about exams or job changes; it can involve less accessible anxieties, such as fears of "letting go" and of death; it can be a mounting prepsychotic anxiety heralding a psychotic episode in a schizophrenic or borderline patient. Obviously, different treatments are required for these different causes.

Among middle-aged and older people, depression is an extremely frequent cause of insomnia. At times the patient may not be experiencing conscious sadness or hopelessness, or may be unwilling to speak of it. In such situations a probable diagnosis of depression can sometimes be made on the basis of insomnia (difficulty in remaining asleep) combined with symptoms such as weight loss, constipation, loss of energy, loss of interest in the world.

There are many environmental causes of insomnia. Obviously noisy or disturbing sleeping environments can produce difficulty in sleep. One of the interesting and quite frequent causes of insomnia is jet-lag. In this condition, the obvious problem is that the body is asked to go to sleep at a time which is appropriate according to local clock-time, but not according to the body's continuing cycles. Luckily this condition usually cures itself within a few days. However, there are occasional severe insomniacs who appear to have a sort of "jet-lag" without having traveled. It appears that their body cycles may be out of phase with one another, for unknown reasons.

There is also a condition sometimes called "habit insomnia." Here the assumption is that whatever causes may have originally produced the insomnia in the past, it is currently maintained by habit or association: the patient's bed is experienced as a place for tossing and turning, a place for insomnia rather than as a place for sleep. Possible treatments of these conditions will be discussed below.

It is not always easy to determine when insomnia is severe enough to require concern or treatment. No quantitative rules can be given. Many people sleep 5 to 6 hours per night and function well, whereas for others this limited sleep duration appears to produce impaired functioning. Some people always take 30 to 60 minutes to fall asleep and enjoy this period of relaxation, while others panic if they are not asleep in 15 minutes. Older people normally have several awakenings each night and these increase with age: for some this is accepted as part of aging, while others see it as a problem requiring treatment. My own view is that there is cause for concern if—and only if—the insomnia or lack of sleep itself clearly interferes with waking activity or mood.

I have not attempted to assign a frequency to the different causes of insomnia. Among insomniac patients I have seen myself and studied in my laboratory, the "psychiatric" causes, especially depression and the several kinds of anxiety discussed, have been the most common. However, this is partly because I am a psychiatrist and am associated with several psychiatric hospitals, so that I do not see a random sample of patients with insomnia. Other researchers have seen very different kinds of patients (see References). For instance, one sleep disorder center reports that a large proportion of its patients have sleep apnea and nocturnal myoclonus. General practitioners usually report that pain or discomfort from chronic illness is a very frequent cause of insomnia in their practices. Thus, I feel that we do not at present truly know the frequency of different causes of insomnia, and it would only be confusing to provide numbers from the sample I have seen.

LABORATORY SLEEP RECORDINGS

Sleep laboratories have now recorded all-night sleep patterns of numerous insomniac patients (see References for some detailed reports). The findings are that, as expected, many insomniacs take longer to get to sleep than normal subjects and many spend more time awake after sleep onset. However, this is by no means always the case. A sizable number of people complaining of insomnia have sleep latencies (time spent getting to sleep) and total sleep times within the normal range. This has given rise to the term *pseudoinsomnia*, discussed below. In addition, many but not all insomniacs can be shown to have a greater than normal number of awakenings, a greater than normal number of shifts between stages, and often less D-sleep than normal sleepers.

Some specific groups have been studied in detail. For instance, most hospitalized depressed patients studied in the laboratory do have very poor sleep, characterized by frequent awakenings during the night, early-morning awakenings, little stage 4 sleep, and many shifts in stages.

One small group of insomniacs has been identified who regularly wake during D-periods. Other groups have somewhat unusual qualitative EEG patterns—for instance, the continuation of waking alpha rhythms throughout sleep. Another group may exist that has less than normal amounts of sleep rhythms, such as the 13 to 15-per-second sleep spindle rhythm or sensorimotor rhythms.

The significance and specificity of these differences is not yet clear, but obviously sleep laboratory studies will help to delineate and characterize subgroups among the insomnias.

"PSEUDOINSOMNIA"

Doctors and sleep researchers sometimes use the term *pseudoinsomnia*. They mean by this that a patient complains of insomnia, of hardly sleeping at all, and yet careful observation by nurses in the hospital or laboratory sleep evaluation reveals that sleep does occur—quite often, four to eight hours of sleep per night. We have certainly found this to be the case at times, and there is absolutely no question that many insomniacs overestimate the time they spend awake and underestimate the time they spend asleep, especially when there have been a number of awakenings during the night. However, we have some preliminary data showing that normal persons who wake up several times during the night for periods of 10 to 15 minutes likewise almost always overestimate the time they spent awake. This is hardly surprising: obviously we are aware of the passage of time when we lie in bed awake but are not aware, or much less aware of it when we are asleep. Therefore I do not believe we should label people who thus overestimate their waking as "pseudoinsomniacs" in the sense of somehow being cheaters or malingerers.

There are, of course, occasional hypochondriacs who tend to

exaggerate all symptoms tremendously for various psychological reasons. However, I believe it is necessary to examine each case individually. If a patient says, "I feel awful, I hardly slept all night," yet the polygraph indicates that he or she slept five hours, or even six to seven hours with a number of awakenings (thus "objectively," not a severe insomnia), it is quite possible that in some senses the patient may be more correct than the polygraph. He is underestimating his sleep time, yet he did wake up frequently during the night, and although he slept five to seven hours, the sleep may not have been of the usual "quality," or sufficient for this particular person.

We know little about exactly what characteristics of a night's sleep are associated with "sleep quality" in the sense of producing a well-rested feeling the next day or adequate daytime functioning. Our laboratory and others have found some trends—feeling good in the morning was related to few awakenings during the night and to more D-time—but the relationships were not strong. Sleep deprivation and sleep reduction studies show that reducing sleep to four or five hours per night for several weeks was associated with problems in motivation (in performing dull tasks), while reducing sleep to two hours per night clearly reduced *ability to perform tasks*. We cannot be sure that the many variables we are able to measure in polygraphic recordings—sleep length, stages of sleep, etc.—are even consistently related to other probably important measures such as "depth" of sleep. In normal subjects, the arousal threshold (intensity of a stimulus needed to awaken) is higher in stages 3–4 than in stages 1–2, and there is some consistency across subjects in arousal threshold. However, this may not be the case in the insomniac. In fact, there is evidence that in depressed patients, normal-appearing stage 2 is not as deep—in terms of arousal threshold—as it is in other people. Thus, there may well be something wrong with the insomniac's sleep despite the fairly normal recorded total sleep time. We may simply not yet know how to detect the important differences.

THE PATHOPHYSIOLOGY
OF INSOMNIA

It is clear from the above that insomnia is not an illness but a symptom or a final common path that can be produced by many different underlying conditions or causes. The mechanisms by which such conditions can produce insomnia are only beginning to be elucidated (fig. 6.1). There are wakefulness or arousal systems within the ascending reticular activating system (ARAS), originating chiefly in the mesencephalon and pons. Some or all of the neurons involved in these arousal systems are dopaminergic or noradrenergic neurons. Thus, conditions associated with increased activation of the ARAS—for instance peripheral pain, muscle spasms, etc.—probably produce insomnia through their effect on the ARAS; and drugs such as amphetamines, which act by releasing and preventing the re-uptake of dopamine and norepinephrine at brain synapses, probably have their effect on the same catecholaminergic systems.

There are sleep systems in the brain, incompletely understood but involving serotonergic neurons with their cell bodies in the raphe nuclei of the brainstem. There is also evidence that certain areas in the medial forebrain are involved in the maintenance of sleep; these neurons are apparently not serotonergic. Insomnias related to neurological lesions of the brainstem may damage this sleep system. Insomnia related to depression may well involve malfunction of the serotonergic systems. The biology of endogenous depression is thought to involve a reduction of functional biogenic amines at certain brain synapses. The catecholamines are certainly involved, but some depressed patients may have abnormalities at serotonin synapses as well; since brain serotonin plays an important role in the mechanism of sleep, it seems likely to me that the depressed patients with severe insomnia may be those who have problems at serotonin synapses. This is being investigated but has not been established as yet.

Figure 6.1 is an attempt to delineate a pathophysiology of insomnia; at this point it involves a great deal of speculation.

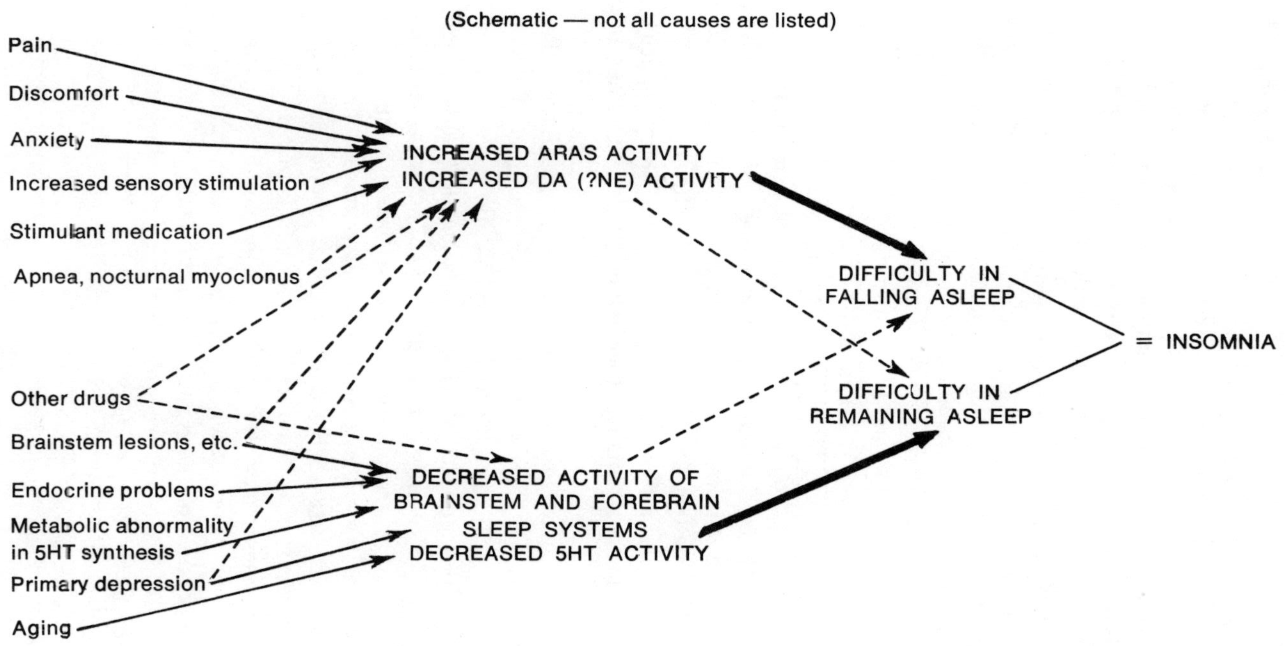

(Schematic — not all causes are listed)

Pain
Discomfort
Anxiety
Increased sensory stimulation
Stimulant medication
Apnea, nocturnal myoclonus

Other drugs
Brainstem lesions, etc.
Endocrine problems
Metabolic abnormality in 5HT synthesis
Primary depression
Aging

INCREASED ARAS ACTIVITY
INCREASED DA (?NE) ACTIVITY

DECREASED ACTIVITY OF BRAINSTEM AND FOREBRAIN SLEEP SYSTEMS
DECREASED 5HT ACTIVITY

DIFFICULTY IN FALLING ASLEEP

DIFFICULTY IN REMAINING ASLEEP

= INSOMNIA

FIGURE 6.1 A Possible Pathophysiology of Insomnia

I do not believe such a scheme is necessary at present in the *clinical* evaluation and treatment of insomnia; however, the scheme may have theoretical implications. For instance, it suggests that certain inborn or acquired brain or metabolic abnormalities will be associated with insomnia. Thus, the patient with "agrypnia," or almost total insomnia, referred to at the end of this chapter apparently had a problem at the tryptophan hydroxylase step in serotonin synthesis. Other problems in the synthesis or metabolism of serotonin, dopamine, and norepinephrine could likewise cause insomnia, as could problems involving the "morphine receptors." Some chronic insomnias could be caused by actual anatomical abnormalities or lesions involving the brainstem.

Many others of the body's endocrine systems could influence sleep indirectly by their effects on the above systems, which I see as playing a primary role. For instance, steroids and insulin can both affect brain serotonin levels; the sex hormones have a complex interrelationship with brain norepinephrine and dopamine; and many other relationships are under investigation.

It is also quite probable that some people have other abnormalities in their body chemistry or metabolism which can interfere with their sleep in ways we do not yet understand. In these persons, specific restoration of chemical balance could be useful. For instance, two patients have described to me a great improvement in their insomnia after taking magnesium salts. Unless this was purely a chance effect, it at least suggests the possibility that electrolyte balance including levels of calcium and magnesium, known to be important for neuromuscular function, is important to normal and abnormal sleep. Much of this, of course, is speculative; hardly any cases of these suggested abnormalities have been carefully studied. We are only beginning to elucidate the pathophysiology of insomnia.

THE TREATMENT OF INSOMNIA

The above discussion must make it obvious that the first step in treating insomnia is a careful medical and psychiatric evaluation. When the diagnosis is not clear on the basis of a clinical evaluation, several nights of sleep in a sleep laboratory or specialized sleep-disorders clinic may be recommended. Conditions such as sleep apnea, nocturnal myoclonus, and a few others can only be clearly demonstrated in the sleep laboratory; and, in addition, sleep patterns in depression are now becoming so well established that sleep laboratory recordings can sometimes help make a diagnosis of endogenous depression when it is not clear on clinical grounds.

The specific treatment will therefore vary with the particular illness or condition producing insomnia. The painful or uncomfortable conditions listed in the first column of table 5.1 will often be amenable to appropriate medical or surgical treatment. Sleep apnea is sometimes found to be secondary to local pathology of the neck and throat, especially of the pharynx. In these cases, a tracheotomy, which can be left open at night to insure proper breathing and closed in the daytime, has often provided dramatic relief. In cases where apnea is due to obesity of local tissues, dieting can also be useful. In instances where sleep apnea appears to be related to a brainstem abnormality ("central type"), stimulant medication is usually the only treatment available.

There is no specific treatment for nocturnal myoclonus at present, though a number of medications can occasionally help. A rare case of nocturnal epilepsy can be treated with antiepileptic medication. In some patients we have seen, myoclonic muscle jerks occur only when patients lie in a certain position. Here a simple mechanical treatment has been useful—namely, arranging beds and pillows in such a way as to make sleep in that position impossible. Sometimes simply reassuring the patient that myoclonus is not a dangerous condition can be extremely useful and can decrease the associated awakenings, even if the actual muscle jerks are not significantly reduced.

When an insomniac patient is taking multiple medications for different causes, it can frequently be suspected that one of the medications, or an interaction between medications, is responsible for the insomnia. Treatment involves carefully withdrawing the medications one by one; it is surprising how often this is successful.

Insomnia that is secondary to psychiatric or environmental conditions also frequently responds to specific treatment. When anxiety of a psychotic or prepsychotic type is responsible for the insomnia, antipsychotic medication is indicated and psychotherapy may also be useful. Anxiety relating to particular conflicts—for instance, anxiety about letting go and losing control of one's aggressive or sexual impulses—is often amenable to specifically oriented psychotherapy. When the problem is chronic and forms a part of the patient's character, long-term nondirective psychoanalysis may sometimes be useful. In some cases of anxiety, antianxiety medications (minor tranquilizers) are helpful as well. In cases where the anxiety is partly muscular, techniques such as relaxation therapy, meditation, or biofeedback can be effective. (These techniques sometimes help other insomniacs as well.) In cases where environmental problems or schedules produce insomnia, a careful evaluation will usually reveal some way in which the environmental factors can be altered.

In primary or endogenous depression, an antidepressant medication will usually improve the insomnia along with the depression. We have found that amitriptyline is the antidepressant medication of choice in a large number of cases. As mentioned above, sometimes insomnia—specifically, difficulty in remaining asleep—occurs in conjunction with other somatic symptoms of depression such as lack of energy, loss of appetite, loss of libido, etc., without any psychological depression (sadness); these cases, nonetheless, often respond well to antidepressant medication such as amitriptyline. Some depressed patients have been reported to have improved dra-

matically after taking l-tryptophan, either alone or in addition
to the more usual antidepressants. We are investigating
whether this subgroup reports insomnia as an especially
prominent symptom (see chap. 10).

I have not tried to describe all possible treatments, but I
hope the main point of the above discussion is clear: a careful
evaluation and specific diagnosis of the cause of insomnia
will in most cases suggest a specific treatment, so that an
illness rather than the symptom insomnia will be treated.

Even when no certain, treatable cause of insomnia can be
determined, there are some simple nonpharmacological treatments that should be tried before turning to long-term use of
sleeping medication. These include careful attention to dietary
intake—there are people who are especially sensitive to the
effects of certain foods. Difficulty in sleeping after drinking
coffee, tea, or some carbonated beverages is common, and
these can be avoided in the evening. Alcohol in very small
doses may help certain people get to sleep, but the pharmacological effects of alcohol are quite disruptive to sleep, and
some insomniacs can definitely benefit from not drinking
any alcohol, or at least avoiding alcohol in the evening.

Exercise may often be useful in moderate quantities, very
regularly, and preferably in the afternoon or early evening
(not immediately prior to bedtime). In people whose bed-
times, mealtimes, and worktimes vary considerably, simply
regularizing one's schedule can considerably improve sleep if
done carefully over a period of weeks or more. Some patients
have developed a vicious cycle or "habit insomnia" (see
above), in which they associate their bed with sleeplessness
instead of sleep: they lie in bed growing increasingly tense
about not getting to sleep, cannot, of course, get to sleep
feeling this way, and so become even more tense, and so on.
In such cases, a form of deconditioning is useful: the patient
is instructed to associate his bed *only with sleep*. If he cannot
get to sleep after five minutes, he is to get out of bed, read a
book, or perform some other activity in another room until
he is worn out and really wants to sleep. He can then return

to bed, but must get up again if he does not fall asleep in a
few minutes, and so on. As can be imagined, this procedure
can be quite painful for a few days, but it has been successful
in helping some severe cases of insomnia.

Do Sleeping Pills Have a Place in the Treatment of Insomnia?

We have seen that many spe-
cific illnesses or conditions can produce insomnia, and whenever possible these causes should be specifically treated. Does
this mean that sleeping pills should never be used? I would
suggest that there are several groups of insomniacs who may
require sleeping pills. Certainly patients with pain or discomfort from medical and surgical conditions will sometimes require sleeping medication for a brief period. Similarly, persons
with insomnia related to environmental changes—changes in
occupation, jet lag, etc.—who are very unhappy about the loss of
a few nights' sleep may sometimes require medication. Patients
with such conditions can be given sleeping pills for a period
of days or weeks, with the understanding of both patient and
doctor that this is to be a short-term measure and that there
may be a period of difficult sleep upon withdrawal of medication.

Long-term use of sleeping pills should be restricted to a
fairly small group of patients who have severe insomnia for
which no clear medical or psychiatric cause has been established, or perhaps when a cause has been established but no
adequate or specific treatment has been found. Since hypnotics
often lose their effectiveness with time, only a subgroup of
these patients probably benefit; we would have to specify
that only the subgroup actually shown to sleep better or
function better on long-term hypnotics should be so treated.
The number of such patients will gradually diminish as new
causes and treatments for insomnia are discovered.

Anyone prescribing or taking sleeping pills should know

that there are certain medical situations in which the administration of a hypnotic can be very dangerous. For instance, in patients with the rare metabolic illness porphyria, the administration of barbiturates can be dangerous and life-threatening. In patients with sleep apnea, where respiratory function is borderline in any case, the additional respiratory depression produced by *any* CNS depressant can be life-threatening.

Likewise, physicians and patients should realize that most hypnotic medications not only lose their effectiveness after long-term administration, but sometimes may actually worsen sleep when they are taken for long periods. In other words, sleeping pills sometimes actually *produce* insomnia through unknown mechanisms. This may sound paradoxical, but it is by no means a theoretical or academic point. It is frequently clinically relevant, especially in cases where multiple medications are being taken together. When I see a patient complaining of serious insomnia and hear that he or she is taking five or six different medications including sleeping pills, I can nearly always be of help by trying carefully to eliminate unnecessary medications one by one. Often to everyone's surprise, the patient then sleeps considerably better without medication. Unfortunately, however, it often takes at least weeks and occasionally months for the effects of previous medication to wear off.

The main point of this chapter is that insomnia is not an illness in itself, but a symptom of a number of different illnesses or underlying conditions. Often these underlying conditions can be identified and a specific treatment applied. The sleeping pill has a relatively restricted place in the treatment of insomnia.

A Note on "Total Insomnia"

I shall briefly discuss here the question of total sleeplessness, whether it be the ability to function without sleep or total inability to sleep, since people often feel that in terms of its semantic roots, *insomnia* really means "no sleep." Total insomnia is an almost unknown condition. Although every year the popular literature comes up with a case of a man in Australia or Italy who got along without sleep, it is usually impossible to locate the person involved, or it turns out that the reports all refer to the same person who died many years ago, making it difficult to verify the situation now.

In fact, researchers who have tried to examine the phenomenon of short sleep—people who can get along well on a few hours of sleep—usually have great difficulty finding subjects. Jones and Oswald, in 1968, reported on three short sleepers who slept approximately three hours a night. Recently, Meddis has reported on several extreme short sleepers of this type who claim to get along on no sleep, or perhaps one hour a night. These have yet to be studied carefully in the laboratory. In our own studies, carried out in our laboratory in Boston and Dr. Baekeland's in New York, we spent over a year searching for a group of subjects who regularly slept less than six hours. We did find a sizable group who, to begin with, claimed that they got along on three to four hours of sleep most of the time. However, when studied extensively in the laboratory, we found that the group of "short sleepers" averaged almost five and one-half hours of sleep, and that none slept less than four and one-half hours. The studies above refer to "short sleep" and not to *insomnia* as we defined it at the beginning of this chapter. Insomniacs studied clinically may complain of "no sleep at all" but seldom sleep less than four to five hours a night over long periods.

There are a few exceptions, however. The neurological literature contains a description of total insomnia lasting for long periods of time in encephalitis (Von Economo in 1929 and 1939) and in conditions known as fibrillary chorea and acrodynia.

There is only one person studied extensively in the laboratory who seemed to qualify as obtaining almost no sleep. This case was described by Fisher-Perroudon in 1973. A young man of twenty-seven had an illness characterized by abdominal pain with diarrhea, burning sensations in his extremities, nighttime sweating, fever, and inability to sleep. The illness developed over several months with increasing fibrillation of all his muscles, extreme burning and pricking pain as well as itching, a rash, episodes of sweating, nocturnal hallucinations, and almost total inability to sleep. He was diagnosed as having the rare condition fibrillary chorea. This patient slept hardly at all over a period of six months, as confirmed in a hospital by nurses' observations and a large number of all-night polygraphic recordings. It is interesting that despite this almost total lack of sleep, the patient was relatively normal during the day and was able to function well on many psychological tests.

However, he was unhappy about his lack of sleep and suffered from two kinds of hallucinations. One kind lasted 20 to 60 minutes every evening and felt somewhat like dreams, with recurring themes that involved a voyage to the moon and a pheasant hunt. The second kind consisted of episodes of "microhallucinations," lasting usually less than a minute but occurring ten to fifty times per night. This man's sleep had not been improved by any known methods and was not helped by sleeping pills. In accordance with our knowledge of the involvement of serotonin in the biochemistry of sleep, this patient was treated with large doses of l-tryptophan and 5-hydroxytryptophan. These substances, especially l-tryptophan, produce sleepiness and reduced time in falling asleep in normal persons (see chap. 10). But on this particular patient l-tryptophan had no effect, while 5-hydroxytryptophan did produce several hours of sleep per night. Because of this, it was felt that the patient had some problem with hydroxylation of tryptophan in the brain.

The patient died after several months in the hospital, and the autopsy did not reveal a specific cause of death. This particular man did sleep extremely little, and the causes are not yet understood, but in his case this was obviously part of an illness. Thus, his case cannot be taken to mean that sleep is not really necessary for us, although some have tried to in-

terpret it this way. In general, cases of almost total insomnia
are almost totally nonexistent, and to the best of my current
knowledge, absolute insomnia is absolutely nonexistent.

References

Bootzin, R. R., and P. M. Nicassio. Behavioral Treatments for In-
somnia. In Hersen, M.; R. Eisler; and P. Miller, eds. *Progress in
Behavior Modification*, vol. 4. New York: Academic Press, in
press.
Dement, W. C. *Some Must Watch While Some Must Sleep.* San
Francisco: W. H. Freeman, 1974.
Fischer-Perroudon, C. Insomnie totale pendent plusieurs mois et
metabolisme de la serotonine. Lyon: Imprimerie Des Beaux-
Arts, 1973.
Greenberg, R. Dream interruption insomnia. *J. Nerv. Ment. Dis.*
144:18–21, 1967.
Guilleminault, C.; F. L. Eldridge; and W. C. Dement. Insomnia
with sleep apnea: A new syndrome. *Science* 181 (1973): 856–
58.
Guilleminault, C.; A. Tilkian; and W. C. Dement. The sleep apnea
syndromes. *Ann. Rev. Med.* 27 (1976): 465–84.
Hartmann, E. Sleep requirement: Long sleepers, short sleepers,
variable sleepers, and insomniacs. *Psychosomatics* 2 (1973): 95–
103.
———. Sleep and Sleep Disorders. In *Handbook of Biological Psychiatry.* New York: Marcel Dekker, 1978 (in press).
———. Drugs for Insomnia. Rational Drug Therapy 11 (1977):
1–6.
Hartmann, E.; F. Baekeland; and G. R. Zwilling. Psychological
differences between long and short sleepers. *Arch. Gen. Psychiat.*
26 (1972): 463–68.
Hauri, P. The Sleep Disorders (Current Concepts). Kalamazoo,
Mich.: Upjohn, 1977.
Hawkins, D. R., and J. Mendels. Sleep disturbance in depressive
syndromes. *Am. J. Psychiatry* 123 (1966): 682–90.
Jones, H. S., and I. Oswald. Two cases of healthy insomnia.
Electroenceph. Clin. Neurophysiol. 24 (1968): 378–80.

Kales, A., and J. D. Kales. Sleep Disorders. *New Eng. J. of Medicine* 290 (1974): 487–99.

Karacan, I., and R. L. Williams. The relationship of sleep disturbances to psychopathology. In Hartmann, E., ed. *Sleep and Dreaming.* International Psychiatry Clinics, vol. 7, no. 2, pp. 93–111. Boston: Little Brown, 1970.

Luce, G. G., and J. Segal. *Insomnia.* New York: Doubleday, 1969.

McFarland, R. A. Air Travel across Time Zones. *Amer. Scientist* 63 (1975): 23–30.

Meddis, R. On the functions of sleep. *Anim. Behav.* 23 (1975): 676–91.

Oswald, I. Sleep and its disorders. *Handbook Clin. Neurol.* 3 (1969): 80–111.

Rechtschaffen, A., and J. Monroe. Laboratory studies of insomnia. In Kales A., ed. *Sleep: Physiology and Pathology,* pp. 158–69. Philadelphia: J. B. Lippincott, 1969.

Von Economo, C. Die Encephalitis lethargica. Ihre Nachrankheiten und ihure Behandlung. Berlin: Urban and Schwarzenberg, 1929.

Zung, W. W.; W. P. Wilson; and W. E. Dodson. Effect of depressive disorders on sleep EEG responses. *Arch. Gen. Psychiat.* 10 (1964): 439–45.

7

The Psychodynamics of the Sleeping Pill

Why do people take sleeping pills? We generally assume people take them because they have trouble sleeping; I can hardly argue that this statement is false, yet the truth is larger and more complex than it implies.

First of all, we have seen that insomnia is a symptom produced by a great number of different medical and psychological causes, many of which have their own specific, appropriate treatments; nonetheless, a huge number of sleeping pills are prescribed for insomnia which has such treatable causes. It seems that most sleeping medications lose their effectiveness, or much of it, after a few weeks of administration; yet a tremendous number of people continue to take the medications for months or years, or even for their entire lives. We have seen that the over-the-counter sleeping pills are in most cases just barely effective, and they do carry some risks; yet a huge number of people go to their drugstores and buy these products. We can also easily find a number of people taking sleeping pills who do not have insomnia at all—perhaps they have some aches or problems or worries, sometimes associated with a bit of trouble getting to sleep—no more than the rest of us—yet they also take medication. Why do all these people take sleeping pills?

We must obviously enlarge our statement: people do not take sleeping pills simply because they have insomnia, but because they ask for sleeping pills (at their physician's office or their drugstore) and someone supplies them. In other words, taking a sleeping pill is an interaction. It is a sociological phenomenon that must have psychological roots. Let us explore some of the reasons, other than obtaining the ideal treatment for an illness, why people may take sleeping pills.

THE COMPLAINT

First, we can consider the symptom or complaint itself. "I have trouble sleeping" sounds simple, but I believe this simple statement both condenses and conceals a set of complex human dynamics. Almost all the "ills that flesh is heir to" may be involved in this complaint, as long as the ills are of a mild or moderate severity. There are thousands of situations in which the patient may sense something like: "I have been feeling uncomfortable ever since my operation; however, I do not think this is really serious and I do not want the doctor to give me a series of complicated tests. Perhaps if I could get something to make me sleep, everything else would improve"; or something like: "I know I have been feeling low and somewhat anxious since my children left home. Perhaps I should talk to a psychiatrist or counselor about it, but that can take a long time and costs money. Besides, I do not want someone digging up my whole past life. Perhaps if I just slept a little better, I would feel more relaxed in the morning and my whole day would be better."

Situations like these are obviously common, and I consider the complaint "I have trouble sleeping" a shorthand expression for them. Most often, the doctor consciously or unconsciously agrees with the patient, or may think something like, "I know it is a painful period for you; I suppose we could do a series of diagnostic studies, but they probably would not demonstrate anything," or "This is obviously a hard time for you. But neither of us has the time or energy to go into it in detail. I think with time you will pull through." The doctor's shorthand response, condensing all these thoughts, is to prescribe a sleeping pill. Sometimes this is the best thing he can do; sometimes, further exploration would be fruitful.

A complaint of insomnia is thus a handy shorthand or

condensation. In addition, it is a convenient and very common symptom, easy to acknowledge and discuss; a patient with many concerns or anxieties may select a sleep problem as the simplest, most acceptable, or easiest one to talk about. Perhaps all this is related to the fact that some degree of insomnia is almost universal—apparently the transition from waking to sleep is a vulnerable point both physiologically and psychologically. We all have a sort of Achilles' heel at this delicate daily transition point.

THE PATIENT

Let us consider in more detail what may be going on with the patient, the doctor, and their interaction. For the patient, there is first of all a simple economic aspect: it is considerable trouble in terms of both time and money to go to a physician, or perhaps to several physicians and psychotherapists, to have a condition carefully evaluated and treated. It is relatively easy, on the other hand, to diagnose oneself—to say, "I am not sleeping well. Perhaps everything else would go better if I got more sleep, so let's try a sleeping pill." Indeed this is, in principle, a perfectly reasonable approach if the patient has mild symptoms and if there is no reason to suspect deep medical or psychological causes of his insomnia. (Of course, the problem is that some of the causes are not easy for the patient himself to suspect.) And it is reasonable to try one of many nondrug aids to sleep, or to take, for a brief time, one of the over-the-counter sleep aids if one is willing to follow the advice on the label that says something like, "If symptoms persist, consult a physician."

Then, if things have gone beyond this point and the patient actually goes to his physician's office, there is again a considerable factor of expense and time. The patient wants help quickly without the expense, trouble, and pain that complex diagnostic procedures or long probing interviews may involve. The physician also has various reasons for his actions.

These are partly matters of time and expense. He probably
has other patients waiting, is rushed, and wants to save his
patient money; or perhaps he has decided after careful consideration that there is little likelihood the patient has specific
medical or psychological problems. Actually, however, it takes
a rare ability to be able to make such an appraisal in only a
few minutes.

What I have discussed so far takes place on a relatively
conscious and rational level. Frequently there is a great deal
more going on. For instance, the patient is asking for help in
one of many ways. He may be saying he has trouble dealing
with competition in the real world or with his competitive
strivings ("I can't take this rat race"). He may be asking for
love and attention ("No one seems to care for me anymore,
Doctor"); expressing loneliness or depression ("I just lie in
bed thinking how nice things used to be and how it's all
gone"); or perhaps expressing helplessness ("I just can't
cope"). Frequently the patient is also asking for an ally ("No
one at home believes me. No one appreciates how hard my
life is").

Complaining of insomnia and obtaining a sleeping pill
frequently involve some of our most primitive psychological
defense mechanisms. Sometimes there is a massive denial that
anything is wrong besides a problem with sleep. Some people
project all that is bad or uncomfortable in their lives onto
sleeplessness, and correspondingly, everything good and helpful is magically projected onto the sleeping pill.

The insomnia itself, and the request for help, can present
problems deriving from every stage of the patient's development. In terms of the psychosexual stages outlined by psychoanalysis, there are sometimes overwhelming oral anxieties:
"I need something I'm not getting; I can't cope; Help!" And,
more concretely, "Give me something to put in my mouth";
or an underlying sense that "no one has fed me right in the
past; I haven't gotten what I needed; now this pill will make
up for it." There is sometimes an anal compulsive element in
forcing oneself to go to sleep: "I've *got* to do it, I've *got* to.";

and tense phallic striving: "I have to be good at everything. I've got to be the best at getting to sleep as well as best at waking activities!"

There is also a type of insomnia that clearly derives from disturbance by id impulses: "I'm afraid to let go or I will kill someone, or be killed myself; or rape someone, or be raped". Sometimes there is a more primitive fear of losing control of reality, merging with someone else, or total disintegration. Or else a conflict with the superego torments the sleeper (as in Macbeth's insomnia).

Obtaining a sleeping pill can temporarily fulfill or appear to fulfill many of these needs or partly overrule these fears. It can mean obtaining permission from an internalized parent who says, "It's all right to go to sleep"; it can be a forgiveness for transgressions. The pill can be a transitional object—like the security blanket a child carries with him to remind himself of home and safety. It is a sign that the doctor, ally, parent, is somehow present and so the patient need not fear his loneliness or helplessness so much.

There is a basic need to prove that one is not worthless: "Someone will give me something to show his love, to show me that I am worth something." Father, mother, uncle, or Santa Claus are summoned up and the sleeping pill becomes a gift, a token of love. The pill can also be an ally against the cruel, uncaring world, much as addicts consider their "shot" or pill or cigarette to be a magical ally or friend. Perhaps all of us are in part addicts and have such needs at certain times. It is very human, and yet somehow very sad, that a breathing, living person must regularly seek a friend in a cigarette, a glass of whiskey, or a sleeping pill. I have discussed the dynamics operative in getting or taking a sleeping pill. In some people there are, of course, also dynamic factors that produce a fear of taking a sleeping pill—or any pill. For instance, a person with a great fear of loss of control may be terrified that any pill will further weaken his already weak control over himself.

THE DOCTOR

The physician, of course, has his or her own psychology which helps to determine the response. We all want to be saviors to some extent, and to help our fellow man. The doctor wants this more than most; it is often a major psychological reason for his choice of profession. For many, to be a good doctor means to be (more or less) all-knowing and all-powerful. It is important for him to show himself and his patient that he knows just what is going on and can handle it actively and definitely, although there are obviously numerous occasions when he doesn't and can't. Thus the doctor, too, is in the grip of many dynamic forces. Often he believes, and with a certain emotional and symbolic justification for his belief, that giving the patient something—a pill, a gift of some kind, a token—is being helpful more directly and more firmly than simply providing words of advice or interpretation. The pill seems more real and more powerful than the word.

Suppose one were to say at the end of an interview with a suffering patient, "Well, it appears that you have some problem sleeping; I don't see any definite medical cause for it; it might be useful if you went to see Dr. Blank, had some tests, etc." This sort of ending to an interview, though it may be intellectually honest, leaves a great deal to be desired in terms of fullfilling the many—chiefly unconscious—needs of both patient and doctor. It sounds weak and pallid when compared to the response: "Here, take one of these every night. Be very careful with alcohol; it may affect you more than usual. I'm sure you will be much better soon. Do let me know in a few weeks how you are doing."

The above is one very frequent dynamic factor. There may be many others, depending on the physician's particular personality and style. And, in an overall sense, the doctor as much as the patient prefers to take the effortless shortcut when possible. Advertising by pharmaceutical firms, as well as

138

The Sleeping Pill

medical traditions, often push him to the conclusion that the sleeping pill is such a shortcut.

THE INTERACTION

I have already mentioned, in several contexts, the interaction between patient and doctor; in fact, the whole giving and taking of pills can be studied as a particular species of interaction. In brief outline, we can see some of the following patterns, in addition to those already discussed in relation to fulfilling particular needs of the patient or the doctor.

For instance, the patient is troubled and anxious about a variety of reasonably adult issues. The doctor, perhaps, is similarly troubled and, on top of it, is busy. He feels a pressure to do *something*; he decides, consciously or unconsciously, that reassurance is what is chiefly needed and adds something concrete to make the reassurance more powerful: "Take one of these every night for a few weeks and you'll be a lot better."

Or a patient is suffering, troubled, has various aches and pains, but obviously doesn't want to be sent to a "shrink," or told that it's "all in your head." The patient is saying, subtly: "You don't believe I'm really suffering, do you? You think I'm making it up." The doctor, unsure but wanting to help and perhaps feeling threatened by his own ignorance, answers: "No, No, of course I believe you; here, take these pills."

Or the patient has been seeing the doctor off and on for a long time for a chronic medical or psychological problem. The doctor is leaving on vacation or for some other reason cannot see the patient for a while. The doctor feels a bit guilty about this desertion and supplies a "transitional object": "Take one of these every night while I'm gone—you'll feel better."

Or the patient may be a difficult one, presenting chronic symptoms the doctor cannot diagnose or treat adequately. The doctor may secretly feel, "Why the hell won't you have a pneumococcal pneumonia or something simple I can help you with?" He may prescribe sleeping pills as an angry rejection or as an acknowledgment of his impotence and inability to help. He is saying, in effect: "You might as well try these; I don't think anything is really going to help you."

And then there are the interactions, already alluded to, which are based on deeper needs in the patient, or at times in the doctor. Some patients have a great need to see their doctor as fatherly and omnipotent; often the doctor tries hard to oblige. Occasionally, a female patient craves pills as a substitute for pregnancy—a kind of oral impregnation. A young male patient may see a pill as a way of magically transferring the doctor's potency and strength to himself. Sometimes a patient is looking for a way out, relief from the cares of the world, and wants to take sleeping pills as a form of poison— a slight suicide; the doctor may well feel a bit depressed too, and sympathize.

If a patient returns for further visits, things can become even more complicated, especially if the treatment has not been entirely successful. Say the patient has been taking sleeping medication but is still complaining of the sleeplessness that brought him to the doctor in the first place. The doctor now again has a choice of exploring the background of the insomnia if he wishes, though generally I believe he is less likely to do so at this second opportunity. He and the patient are more likely to assume that the diagnosis was made on the first visit and that it is now merely a matter of adjusting the treatment; all that can be done is to increase the dose or change to another sleeping medication. If this happens a number of times, the patient may become depressed about his lack of improvement, while the doctor frequently grows annoyed and angry at the patient for not responding positively, thus preventing the doctor from fulfilling his role of healer. The doctor may convey his anger subtly or not so subtly to the patient who is, in effect, asked or forced to go and seek help, if he desires it, from another physician; then the whole process may be repeated.

Obviously, I am examining problems that arise and are often overlooked; in other words, I am emphasizing negative possibilities. Sometimes, of course, the pill—combined with all the dynamic forces of the relationship and with the passage of time—has its desired effect; it helps the patient over a difficult period, and eventually the doctor and patient decide it is no longer needed.

The possibilities are numerous. What I am trying to emphasize is that there is a relationship between patient and doctor, even on the first visit. And relationships are not made up of purely rational elements. Even a brief relationship has elements that derive from the past, often from childhood. The emotional elements transferred to a current relationship from past relationships with parents and other important persons are known as "transference." Transference is sometimes thought of as an esoteric, long-term phenomenon—a transfer of feelings specifically from parents to therapist which develops during psychoanalysis or long-term psychotherapy. This is, in fact, true of the full "transference neurosis." However, transference is in the air all the time, for all of us. When we intensely like or dislike someone at first sight, this is often a matter of the conscious or unconscious transference of feelings originally relating to an important person earlier in our lives. (Though it sounds somewhat unkind to mention it, love is often a transference phenomenon.)

A patient comes to a doctor with a whole series of immediate transference feelings and transference expectations. When the doctor is an older adult male, these feelings often relate to the patient's father, or if the doctor is female, to the patient's mother, but many other transference relationships are also possible. And, of course, all this occurs in the other direction as well. The doctor has immediate feelings about the patient, based on his own past, and may also have strong emotional reactions to the patient's transference feelings. These cannot be totally ignored, although they may play a lesser role since the meeting is usually less intense for the doctor.

Thus, in addition to the present-tense psychological factors, irrational echoes from the patient's or the doctor's past also influence the prescribing of a sleeping pill.

RESPONSE TO TREATMENT

We have seen that there are psychological factors involved in producing many sorts of insomnia; we have also seen that psychological factors enter into the demand for a sleeping pill by the patient and the providing of it by the physician. Similar factors affect the results of treatment as well. I believe that all these dynamic factors, plus a number of probable biological variables, all enter into what some have tried to pin down as factors involved in the "drug response." There have been a number of attempts to differentiate statistically different groups of drug responders, or to differentiate "drug responders" from "placebo responders." This aspect of sleep research has recently been reviewed by Beutler and Jobe.* Basically, the conclusion is that it is impossible at this point to predict drug response precisely from what we know of the pharmacology of the drug or the personality of the patient, or both. These factors simply increase the complexity of the situation and help to explain the fact that different persons, when they do require sleeping pills, seem to react quite differently and to be satisfied with very different medications.

CONCLUSIONS

We have seen that obtaining and taking a sleeping pill is a complex human transaction involving many of our basic wishes and needs. Man is a creative as well as a wish-fulfilling animal: when our wishes are not fulfilled in reality, we create dreams to fulfill them. Some create art to express needs and feelings that cannot be acted on directly. When the world is terrifying and unexplainable,

* L. E. Beutler and A. M. Jobe, "Significant Variables in the Psychology and Pharmacology of Sleep," in R. L. Williams and I. Karacan, eds., *Pharmacology of Sleep* (New York: John Wiley & Sons, 1976).

we create gods and demons to make sense of things. I believe we have made a sort of god, or rather a genie-in-a-bottle, out of the sleeping pill: the fulfillment of so many of our deep needs are thus conveniently "encapsulated."

Can anything be done about this? The needs, briefly sketched above, are ubiquitous, and they are crying for fulfillment. They will not disappear simply as a result of a little added knowledge or a few words of explanation like the contents of this chapter. On the other hand, I cannot believe that the result of these intense forces need inevitably be the overuse of sleeping pills.

The forces can at least be recognized and to some extent modified by reality. The doctor can recognize, with effort, some of the forces acting on himself; and, with less effort, many of those affecting the patient. He will see that they are much more powerful in some people than in others. The patient also can, within limits, become wiser. There are obviously some patients who are willing to trust their intellects to a considerable extent and for whom words of advice, or self-understanding, can be worth far more than sleeping pills. The doctor should not underestimate the degree to which he himself, his personality, his spending time with the patient, his perhaps writing down on a piece of paper a few simple suggestions about diet or exercise, coffee or alcohol, will have some of the same symbolic power as the handing over of a prescription.

Yet it is inevitable that a prescription for a sleeping pill will sometimes continue to be useful for emotional rather than for ideally rational and medical reasons; in these cases, the doctor might consider prescribing a placebo or something safe and pharmacologically weak so that possible harmful effects will at least be minimized. Obviously sleeping pills are not about to vanish. But we can attempt to make the substances used in them more rational and safe (see chaps. 9 and 10), and we can at least be aware of all the powerful forces outlined here which make us prescribe and take sleeping pills considerably more often than we should.

8

The Benefits and Risks
of Sleeping Pills

Generally speaking, a drug is made available, is prescribed, and retains a solid place in medical practice when it has found a specific use—for instance, in treating a well-defined illness—and when the benefits of its use prove, by and large, to outweigh the risks. This does not mean that the risks must be few or negligible. An anticancer compound may (and often does) have many severe side effects and risks. These could make it a horrendous drug if it were prescribed for minor ailments or sold over the counter: however, the problems may be acceptable when the medication is administered to a carefully chosen group of patients in whom it has a chance of being a life-saving agent or of prolonging life. (Great risks are sometimes justified by potentially great benefits.) On the other hand, when a drug is prescribed widely in situations where the benefits are small or moderate (relief of headache, cold symptoms, etc.), the risks are expected to be correspondingly small.

The large question of risks and benefits includes broad issues such as "benefits to society," which cannot always be precisely defined or quantified; it also prominently includes the issues of safety and efficacy, which can, to a considerable extent, be examined scientifically. The questions the Food and Drug Administration (FDA) asks of a new drug, or of a drug that has been on the market for some time, are the specific ones of safety and efficacy. Are the drugs reasonably safe? Do they work? For sleeping pills, the answers are not totally encouraging.

What I shall do first is examine the questions of safety and efficacy for the class of hypnotic medication as a whole. I

shall indicate when a drug or group of drugs constitutes an
exception but I shall not try to quantify the safety or effectiveness of specific agents, nor shall I recommend the use or rejection of any individual drugs. I shall then return to the broad
issue of benefits and risks.

SAFETY

The question of safety involves
a number of separate issues, the first and most obvious of
which concerns the direct danger of death, and the lethal dose
of a drug. Most hypnotic drugs have been lethal drugs. They
usually possess a low therapeutic index because they are nonspecific CNS depressants and respiratory depressants. A dose
not too much larger than the therapeutic dose can often result
in coma and death. For instance, the usual effective dose of
secobarbital, the most widely used hypnotic barbiturate, is
100 mg; insomniacs quite often take 200 or 300 mg or even
more at night. Lethal doses are difficult to estimate exactly
because of wide variations between individuals; however, a
fair estimate would be to say that 800 mg can produce coma,
and 2000 to 3000 mg are likely to produce death in a normal
adult. Children, adults having especially low body weight,
adults with various illnesses, and adults taking other depressant
medication can be in danger from considerably lower doses.
Thus, for these drugs, a dangerous dose is not very many times
the usual therapeutic dose.

Overdoses of sleeping pills, especially barbiturates, account
for a large number of deaths. The exact figures are difficult to
determine: it is not always easy to obtain information on the
presence of substances in blood and other tissues, and when
levels *are* reported, one cannot conclude that the mere presence of a substance was necessarily responsible for the death.
When no determinations are obtained, should one rely on a
report by a relative, for example, that the deceased "swallowed
a whole lot of pills"? Obviously some guesswork is involved,
but as a rough guide one source reports that in New York
City alone there were 1,165 fatalities from barbiturate poison-

ing between 1957 and 1963 (Goodman and Gilman, 1970). Another source states that for the country as a whole there are over 15,000 deaths per year directly attributable to sleeping pills, most often barbiturates (Wesson and Smith, 1977). The actual number of deaths is probably larger, since deaths involving suicide or accidents with a possibility of suicide are always underreported.

Since hypnotic medications generally depress all portions of the central nervous system, the mechanism of death is usually respiratory depression. In this respect, most of the recent nonbarbiturates (see chap. 2) resemble the barbiturates. The benzodiazepines constitute an exception; it is almost impossible to kill oneself by taking an overdose of a benzodiazepine.

Another danger or risk involves drug withdrawal. People who take sleeping medication regularly (either by prescription or illegally) often experience serious symptoms on withdrawal. Sudden withdrawal of barbiturates is followed by irritability, insomnia, and occasionally convulsions and death. Unpleasant effects sometimes last for a period of weeks. Some drugs in the nonbarbiturate groups appear to produce fewer problems on withdrawal, but investigation of the more recent compounds is not yet complete. Even the benzodiazepines sometime produce disturbing effects on withdrawal. Often withdrawal symptoms are worse when other medications are being taken simultaneously.

For unknown reasons, the hypnotic drugs have almost invariably been abused. The pharmacological and psychological mechanisms of addiction and abuse are complex and poorly understood, but it is quite striking how often hypnotic medications are implicated.*

* There is room for argument here. The term *abuse* is not clearly defined and is obviously judgmental and pejorative. However, I personally feel that the widespread experimental use, street use, and overuse of powerful sleeping pills must be counted among their serious dangers. This is not because I consider any experimenting with drugs to be evil, but because I have a tendency to favor life over death, health over

[continued on next page]

Another problem derives from the fact that the body rapidly develops tolerance for sleeping pills, so that the original dose is usually no longer effective after a few weeks. This encourages some users to increase the dosage, leading to the dangers we have already discussed.

As a rule, hypnotic medications are foreign substances that are not rapidly metabolized and excreted. The body must greatly increase its enzyme activities and synthesize new enzymes in order to handle the drug.* Thus, either the drug itself or an active metabolite often has a very long half-life in the body. Therefore, even hypnotic medications which are not specifically labeled as long-acting may have "hangover" effects the next day. As we discussed in chapter 5, these after-effects are only beginning to be investigated; however, there is little doubt that tiredness or grogginess the next day does occur and can constitute a danger to someone driving a car or operating machinery.

As with most drugs, there are problems of allergy, hypersensitivity, and interaction with other medications; some of the hypnotic drugs have been especially troublesome in terms of such interactions. For instance, taking barbiturates greatly alters the metabolism and consequently the activity of the most common anticoagulant medications (drugs used to prevent blood clotting); such an interaction can be very dangerous.

The problem is that allergy and hypersensitivity are caused by individual factors impossible to predict, and likewise drug interactions often cannot be predicted ahead of time. As it is not possible to carry out studies on every possible drug interaction, interactions frequently only become known after a

---

illness, whole limbs over broken ones. There is absolutely no question that death, illness, and accidental injury are hugely increased when powerful CNS depressants are at work in the brains of waking (not sleeping) persons who have ready access to various additional depressants such as alcohol and to other marvels of modern technology such as automobiles and handguns.

* These enzymes, in turn, alter the way the body handles other drugs and are responsible for some of the interactions with other drugs.

drug has been in widespread use for a number of years. When proponents of an uncommon or recently introduced drug claim that there are few drug interactions, it is quite conceivable that interactions have simply not yet been discovered.

In a society where alcohol, nicotine, and marijuana are commonly consumed, we should, of course, worry about the interaction* of any other substance with these. However, studies of such interactions are not required before marketing a drug and are seldom conducted at all except when hundreds of adverse reactions have already been reported. Although this is a more general problem not particularly restricted to sleeping pills, some of the commonly used sleeping pills produce especially serious problems of interaction. It is generally acknowledged that one should exercise caution when taking pills along with alcohol, for instance, but I believe the dangers have been underestimated. For example, the benzodiazepines have a very high therapeutic index—a high ratio of lethal dose to therapeutic dose—when taken by themselves, yet I have seen some very disturbing reactions in a few individuals when benzodiazepines were taken simultaneously with moderate amounts of alcohol. These consisted of loss of judgment and an almost psychotic state lasting several hours; in two cases this combination led to serious auto accidents.

It is worth repeating a point I mentioned when discussing the treatment of insomnia in chapter 6. Patients with certain specific physical conditions may be unusually susceptible to the effects of sleeping pills. Patients with porphyria can die from the use of barbiturates; those with sleep apnea may die from the use of any respiratory depressant; and those with serious liver or kidney disease may not metabolize or excrete medication properly and consequently may be in danger from much smaller doses of sleeping pills than most people.

Finally, hypnotic drugs produce a behavioral state resem-

* We are concerned here with risks, and thus with any *clinically dangerous "interaction,"* even though from the strictly pharmacological viewpoint some of these may involve the simple *additive* effect of two depressants.

bling sleep but which is usually not normal sleep by polygraphic criteria: there are clear-cut qualitative and quantitative differences between drug-induced and non-drug sleep,
observable in all-night recordings, as I have discussed in
chapter 5. Admittedly, the clinical significance of these differences is not yet certain, but it is likely that great distortions
of normal sleep patterns, and production of brain-wave patterns that could as easily be called light anesthesia as sleep,
have some meaningful effects. It has not been established that
interfering with or reducing the amounts of any sleep stage
is definitely detrimental, yet I, along with many other sleep
researchers, find it disturbing to see that hypnotic medications
produce regular and long-term changes involving the portions
of sleep considered most important: thus D-sleep (REM
sleep), frequently assigned an important functional role in
the homeostasis of the brain as well as in learning and
memory consolidation, is reduced by most hypnotics. Deep
slow-wave sleep—stage 3 and 4 sleep—is unaffected by many
hypnotics but drastically reduced by the benzodiazepines.
Stage 3 and stage 4 sleep are the other portions of sleep often
thought to be functionally important, perhaps in terms of
protein synthesis or tissue repair. In addition, stage 3 and stage
4 sleep stimulate the daily peak of growth hormone secretion;
reduction of growth hormone secretion might theoretically be
harmful, especially to children. A great deal of further work
is required to determine whether these many possible dangers
have actual clinical relevance.

Are these problems really of serious concern or have I been
exercising my ingenuity in listing as many theoretical problems as possible? Except for the deaths from overdosage,
should the other problems be taken seriously, or are they
"inconveniences" rather than real risks? My belief is that the
risks are real and that the problems listed above produce a
great many deaths and illnesses directly and indirectly; but of
course this statement is not easy to prove.

Some relevant overall data come from a large-scale statis-

tical study carried out by the American Cancer Society. Close
to one million adults, ages thirty to ninety, were asked to fill
out a questionnaire about their health and habits. Among
other things, the questionnaire asked if they ever used sleeping pills. The subjects were followed up to determine who
had died five to ten years later. Those who originally said
they took sleeping pills "often" were 1.5 times as likely to
have died (compared to controls), even when age and hours
of sleep were controlled, and even when persons reporting
high blood pressure, heart disease, stroke, and diabetes were
not considered (Kripke, 1976). These figures are impressive
and highly significant statistically. On the other hand, it must
be remembered that no cause-and-effect relationship between
the use of sleeping pills and the subsequent deaths has been
established. It is quite possible that many of the excess deaths
in the sleeping-pill group were attributable to the many illnesses for which or during which sleeping pills are used,
rather than resulting in any way from the use of medication.

                    The efficacy of sleeping pills
has been discussed to some extent in chapter 5, and I have
mentioned some of the problems and inadequacies in the sleep
studies reviewed. I would say that, generally, efficacy is present
for most hypnotics, but with several important qualifications.
First of all, there are drugs whose effectiveness at clinical dose
levels is in question: for example, there are conflicting opinions
as to whether methapyrilene (the most widely used over-the-
counter drug) is effective at the usual dose of 25 mg or 50
mg. There are also conflicting reports as to the efficacy of 500
mg of chloral hydrate, though there is better evidence in favor
of the frequently used dose of 1000 mg.
    Secondly, although the effectiveness of many drugs has
been demonstrated, their efficacy has been determined only
for one night or for a few consecutive nights of administra-

tion. A study by Kales et al., (1975), found that a number of hypnotics no longer produced beneficial effects on sleep after several weeks of nightly administration. In this study, the benzodiazepine flurazepan did maintain its effectiveness, but this result has yet to be replicated. Few studies are available on truly long-term use of hypnotics, but my impression, from data available as well as from clinical experience, is that a large number of persons who habitually take hypnotic medication are taking it basically to avoid withdrawal symptoms, and not because of continued efficacy. They are probably sleeping no better now than they would have slept without medication.

We have seen that the sleep produced by hypnotic medication differs in many ways from normal sleep, so that even in the cases where efficacy is established, we have to speak of efficacy in producing "behavioral sleep" or "a state resembling sleep."

Finally, it must be kept in mind that even drugs of demonstrated efficacy do not simply "improve sleep" in all respects. Frequently studies have shown efficacy in reducing sleep latency (time getting to sleep) or total waking time, which usually is defined as including sleep latency. Thus, often the effect is a reduction of wakefulness and increase of sleep for only a few hours after administration of the drug. There are few studies demonstrating efficacy of a drug on sleep or wakefulness four to eight hours after administration. (Of course, short duration of action may be an advantage, because relatively long-lasting drugs—some barbiturates and perhaps flurazepan—may be associated with side effects lasting into the next day.)

Thus, taking into account these qualifications, we cannot simply say that sleeping pills are effective. We can fairly state that, in the usual dosage, most but not all sleeping pills are effective, when first administered, in reducing wakefulness and producing a behavioral state resembling sleep for a few hours after administration.

RISKS AND BENEFITS

Judging the overall risks and benefits of a medication is a broader task than investigating its safety and efficacy. One must consider such problematic factors as the seriousness of the condition being treated, the possibility of serious risks and dangers in leaving the condition untreated or treated by other available means, the possibility of other superior treatments available, and so on.

I have served for some years on an advisory panel for the U.S. Food and Drug Administration (FDA) that was asked to perform the task of weighing risks and benefits for a number of individual drugs. I know that making such a decision for an individual drug is often difficult; thus, an attempt to weigh the risks and benefits of an entire class of medications might appear impossible, foolhardy, or somewhat arrogant. To claim scientific validity for such a judgment would, in fact, merit all three of these adjectives. Nonetheless, I shall attempt such an overall decision—a personal judgment which cannot be proven scientifically—because I believe that to come to no decision or conclusion after reviewing all this information would in itself be a decision, a decision in favor of the status quo—a statement that individual drugs and patients are so different, and the whole situation so complicated, that nothing of any general use can be said or done.

The risks of sleeping pills are those enumerated above in my discussion of safety. The benefits are the benefits of a good night's sleep in a person who has been sleeping poorly, and these can be immense. Anyone who has suffered from insomnia can testify that relief from it is a tremendous advantage in terms of ability to work and enjoy life. The curing of insomnia in a surgeon, an airline pilot, a general, or a president could at certain times literally save lives and nations. On a more everyday level, relief from insomnia can often prevent fights, work conflicts, and accidents. I stated above that a certain number of car accidents may be caused partly by the aftereffects of sleeping pills; I must now also mention that sleeping pills probably prevent a number of accidents that might have been caused partly by the after effects of insomnia. I have no way of estimating the exact number on either side.

Thus, there is no question that benefits do exist. However, these are the benefits of a good night's sleep in a well-rested state, and not just the benefits of a sleeping pill. In many instances of insomnia, better treatments exist (chap. 6) and the desired benefit could be produced in an alternative way. In many other cases, as we have seen, the benefits exist but are short-lived; subsequently, the drugs produce little positive benefit but are taken only to avoid the discomfort of withdrawal. Often the seriousness of the condition being treated is in question. While severe insomnia is debilitating and bears careful examination, a large number of persons take sleeping pills for mild or trivial insomnia; some subject themselves to the risk of sleeping pills when they do not have insomnia at all but merely expect that they *might* have trouble sleeping.

Having considered all these factors, let me now, with some trepidation, make a general evaluation. *I believe that the risks of sleeping pills, as sleeping pills have actually been used over the past few decades, outweigh the benefits.* I believe that despite the benefits discussed, sleeping pills have frequently been misused, consistently abused, and generally overused.

Now that I have stated that the overall risks outweigh the benefits, I must in fairness add that this statement is not equally true under all conditions. It is truer for the long-term than the short-term use of sleeping pills, and it is truer of the barbiturate and nonbarbiturate respiratory depressants than of the benzodiazepines. Still, I firmly believe that my general evaluation is true, and I mean it as a statement that all is not well and something needs to be done.

Does this mean that the FDA or some governmental agency should step in and ban sleeping pills as a class? I do not think so, although a case can be made for banning specific drugs or groups of drugs after severe problems have been found. I have indicated that I believe sleeping pills do have a place. I can think of two steps that need to be taken, and I have been making modest efforts to take both of them.

First, information and education are essential. Physicians should be far more aware of the problems and dangers of medications and of possible alternatives so that prescribing a sleeping pill will become fairly infrequent and administration of sleeping pills for a period of years a very rare occurrence. The consumers of sleeping pills also require educating; whether they are considering consulting a physician about insomnia or medicating themselves with over-the-counter drugs, they should at least understand the multiple causes of insomnia and various possibilities for treatment, as well as the temporary nature of many forms of insomnia. Physicians are only human and often have too little time to see a particular patient. It is important that the patient be sufficiently informed so that his attitude will be: "Please help me to find out what is the matter; let's see what we can do about it," rather than a form of pressure on the doctor: "Help! I can't sleep! Quick, give me a pill!". This book is an effort toward such an education.

Second, now that we know a good deal about the basic chemistry and physiology of sleep, it should be possible to develop a safe and "physiological" substance for use in cases where a sleeping pill is still required. Such a substance should be related to normal sleep and not simply be a CNS depressant; consequently, it should not suffer from the many risks and problems discussed above. This approach is pursued in the next chapter.

References

AMA Department of Drugs: AMA Drug Evaluations. Acton, Mass.: Publishing Sciences Group, 1973.
Goodman, L. S., and A. Gilman. The Pharmacological Basis of Therapeutics. 4th ed. London and Toronto: The MacMillan Co., 1970.
Kales, A.; E. O. Bixler; T.-L. Tan; et al. Chronic hypnotic-drug

use. Ineffectiveness, drug-withdrawal insomnia, and dependence. *JAMA* 227 (1974): 513–17.

Kales, A.; J. D. Kales; E. O. Bixler; et al. Effectiveness of hypnotic drugs with prolonged use: Flurazepam and pentobarbital. *Clin. Pharmacol. Ther.* 18 (1975): 356–63.

Kripke, D. F., and R. N. Simons. Average Sleep, Insomnia and Sleeping Pill Use. Sleep Research 5 (1976): 110.

Wesson, D. R., and B. D. E. Smith, *Barbiturates: Their Use, Misuse and Abuse.* New York: Human Sciences Press, 1977.

9

Toward a Safe and Rational Sleeping Pill: Three Approaches

I shall now consider the way sleeping pills have been developed in the past and then suggest some new ways related to the chemistry of sleep that could result in more rational and safer hypnotic agents. I shall discuss several possibilities, concentrating especially on the amino acid l-trytophan.

DRUG DEVELOPMENT

In some areas of medicine, and at times even in psychiatry, rational development of pharmacological agents proceeds along a relatively straight path. For instance, once it had been recognized that certain frequent groupings of mental symptoms occurred together and could be given a diagnostic label of general paresis; when it was recognized that general paresis formed a part of the systemic disease syphilis; and when it was proven that syphilis resulted from infection by a specific organism, treponema pallidum, it was then possible to investigate, in vitro and in vivo, the antitreponemal activity of drugs found useful against other infectious agents. In this way, treatment with penicillin early in the illness was found to prevent the development of general paresis and has helped reduce its incidence to almost zero in many parts of the world. Medicine also affords a great many examples of illnesses in which there is no infectious agent, but where knowledge of the normal biochemistry or endocrinology had led to the findings of specific abnormalities which then allowed a rational search for therapeutic agents.

In other areas, there may be neither evidence of an infectious agent nor thorough understanding of the biochemical basis of a disease, but there may be one or more tenable theories as to changes responsible for an illness which at least suggest approaches for pharmacotherapeutic development. For example, in psychiatry at present, there are theories about the pathophysiology of both major depression and schizophrenia which allow a rational search for therapeutic agents.

In still other areas, drugs have been developed purely empirically, on the basis of an original, perhaps serendipitous finding, with further elaborations of compounds similar to the first one. This approach may be the only one available when neither biochemistry nor pathophysiology of a condition to be treated is known.

Development of hypnotic medications in the past has occurred only on an empirical basis. The accidental discovery of the depressant properties of bromides and of chloral hydrate prompted their widespread use and a search for related compounds. Later, the chance discovery of the depressant properties of barbital led to a new series of compounds. In more recent years, a number of drugs have been discovered through widespread screening by the pharmaceutical industry for substances that would cause mice to lie down ("loss of righting reflex") and by investigating among members of other drug classes specific agents that appeared to have sedative side effects in man. These lines of drug development began without reference to any knowledge of the biochemistry of normal sleep and have continued in recent years as though we still possessed no such knowledge or theory. An entire book appeared recently entitled *Hypnotics: Methods of Development and Evaluation* (Kagan et al., 1974). The work deals with sophisticated methods of preclinical and clinical drug testing and evaluation, but there is not a single word about a rational choice of substances to be tested.

These empirical procedures have resulted in a number of useful hypnotic drugs, but the drugs have been nonspecific

CNS depressants and have been beset with major problems, as we have seen.

I believe that problems and dangers are inevitable so long as we develop and market drugs which possess powerful and generalized depressant properties. I would like to suggest three possible routes that might lead to the development of a rational hypnotic agent and to follow one of the routes a considerable distance, since my laboratory has already completed many relevant studies.

BRAIN PEPTIDES: ENKEPHALINS AND RELATED SUBSTANCES

In the last few years it has been discovered that the brain contains receptors which are sensitive to morphine and similar chemical compounds (Pert, Pasternak, and Snyder, 1973; Pert, 1974). This suggests that the body might contain its own endogenous, morphinelike substances which act on these receptors. In fact, a number of substances that act upon these "opiate receptors" have recently been discovered in the brain as well as elsewhere in the body. These compounds have been given various names. Some of them are referred to as endorphins (endogenous morphines); on chemical analysis they turn out to be peptide chains. Several of the shorter peptide chains are widely distributed in the brain and are now called enkephalins (Chang et al., 1976; Horn and Rogers, 1976). Their exact functions in the body are currently unknown, but a relationship to pain perception is implied by some studies. I suggest that these substances should be of great interest to the field of sleep research because they resemble, and may even include, the sleep factors isolated and studied in the rabbit by Monnier and in the goat by Pappenheimer.

I mentioned briefly, in chapter 4, research concerning sleep-inducing substances found in the body following a period of sleep deprivation. A group led by Pappenheimer in Boston found a substance in the spinal fluid of sleep-deprived goats (but not normal goats) that was able to induce sleep in rats (Pappenheimer et al., 1967, 1975). Monnier and his collaborators in Switzerland have isolated and studied a substance in the blood of sleep-deprived rabbits which induced sleep in normal rabbits (Monnier et al., 1964, 1972; Schoenenberger and Monnier, 1974). These two pieces of work have remained interesting but peripheral aspects of sleep research: both groups have had great trouble purifying and isolating their substances, and the substances tentatively obtained could not subsequently be related to other known aspects of sleep chemistry. Recently, Monnier has reported the exact structure of his substance in the rabbit; the compound is a short peptide consisting of nine amino acids (Monnier and Schoenenberger, 1977). The structure of the goat substance is not yet absolutely certain, but it appears also to be a short peptide chain, consisting of two to five amino acids.

The rabbit substance contains l-tryptophan as one of its terminal amino acids, and it is conceivable that this could be related to its sleep-inducing effects (see chap. 10). However, it is worth investigating the possibility that both peptides are among the endogenous morphinelike substances and that they may act directly at opiate receptors in the brain. It will be important to determine whether the "sleep peptides," like the opiates, have analgesic as well as hypnotic properties.

In any case, the work on the endogenous peptides will certainly be important for sleep research. These compounds, perhaps possessing both analgesic and hypnotic properties, may somehow reduce the sensitivity of brain centers to afferant (incoming) stimuli. Also there are many ways, just beginning to be elucidated, in which brain peptides interact with brain catecholamines and serotonin, which can be relevant to sleep.

Thus, although there is no firm evidence yet, I am suggesting that certain endogenous morphinelike peptide substances may be involved in the natural induction of sleep in the body. From the point of view of my present discussion of sleeping pills, this produces the interesting implication that the oldest known sleeping pills—the much-maligned opium substances—may after all bear a close relationship to certain normal physiological sleep mechanisms. Possibly the development of sleep-inducing peptides, or substances resulting in the release or activation of the naturally occurring peptides, could be one important avenue toward the rational development of sleeping pills. This is an area for future research which has barely been explored.

BRAIN CATECHOLAMINES

A second rational line of investigation concerns the activity of the ascending reticular activating systems (ARAS), which is essential in maintaining wakefulness (Moruzzi and Magoun, 1949). From the chemical point of view, ascending dopaminergic and perhaps also norepinephrine pathways appear to be important in this wakefulness-mediating system (Fuxe et al., 1970). Thus, drugs which either interfere with the synthesis of catecholamines (dopamine and norepinephrine) in the brain, or block their action, could be investigated. Drugs related to methyldopa or alpha-methyl-paratyrosine, which block enzymes necessary for the synthesis of dopamine and norepinephine, could be considered; unfortunately, these two specific drugs have many side effects and problems that make them unsuitable.

A reasonable group of drugs to consider would be the dopamine receptor blockers. In fact, the best-known receptor blockers, the phenothiazines and other antipsychotics, do have some hypnotic potency. In our studies (Appendix A) chlorpromazine decreased wakefulness and tended to increase sleep time. If one examines only sleep laboratory recordings, from our studies and others, chlorpromazine, the most widely used phenothiazine, appears to be an excellent hypnotic agent: both sleep latency and wakefulness are reduced and the sleep stages are not greatly altered. Chlorpromazine does not produce the great reductions in D-time and stage 4-time which are characteristic of sleep after most hypnotics. However, when one examines the subjective reports, problems begin to emerge: nonpsychotic subjects report considerable morning-after tiredness and grogginess after even a small clinical dose (50 mg) of chlorpromazine at night. Possibly an even smaller dose would avoid these effects.

Unfortunately, the phenothiazines have other serious side effects that make them unsuitable for widespread use in treating insomnia. These include rare cases of damage to the liver and bone marrow and more frequent cases of movement disorders (tardive dyskinesia) after prolonged use. Therefore, it would not be justifiable to use them at present except perhaps in some cases of severe chronic insomnia that are untreatable in other ways. However, it is possible that a dopamine receptor blocker could be developed which had few of these side effects and might be of greater use as a hypnotic agent.

A third rational line of investigation, involving the amino acid l-tryptophan, is considered in the next chapter.

References

Chang, J. K.; B. T. W. Fong; A. Pert; and C. B. Pert. Opiate receptor affinities and behavioral effects of enkephalin: structure-activity relationship of ten synthetic peptide analogues. *Life Sci.* 18, no. 12 (1976): 1473–82.

Fuxe, K.; T. Hokfelt; and U. Ungerstedt. Morphological and functional aspects of central monoamine neurons. *Int. Rev. Neurobiol.* 13 (1970): 93–126.

Horn, A. S., and J. R. Rodgers. Structural and conformational relationships between the enkephalins and the opiates. *Nature* 260, no. 5554 (1976): 795-97.

Kagen, F.; T. Harwood; K. Rickels; A. D. Rudzik; and H. Sorer. Hypnotics: Methods of Development and Evaluation. New York: Spectrum Publications, 1974.

Monnier, M.; A. M. Hatt; L. B. Cueni; C. A. Schoenenberger. Humoral transmission of sleep VI. In *Pfluegers Arch.* 331 (1972): 257–65.

Monnier, M., and L. Hosil. Dialysis of sleep and waking factors in blood of the rabbit. *Science* 146, no. 3645 (1964): 796–98.

Monnier, M., and G. A. Schoenenberger. The delta sleep inducing peptide DSIP. Paper presented to the APSS, Houston, Texas, April 1977.

Moruzzi, G., and H. Magoun. Brain stem reticular formation and activation of the EEG. *Electroenceph. Clin. Neurophysiol.* 1 (1949): 455–73.

Pappenheimer, J.; T. Miller; and C. Goodrich. Sleep promoting effects of EST from sleep-deprived goats. *Proc. Natl. Acad. Sci. USA* 58 (1967): 513–17.

Pappenheimer, J. R.; G. Koski; V. Fencl; M. L. Karnovsky; and J. Krueger. Extraction of sleep-promoting factor S from cerebrospinal fluid and from brains of sleep-deprived animals. *J. Neurophysiol.* 38, no. 5 (1975): 1299–1311.

Pert, C. B.; D. Aposhian; and S. H. Snyder. Phylogenetic distribution of opiate receptor binding. *Brain Res.* 75, no. 2 (1974): 356–61.

Pert, C. B.; G. Pasternak; and S. H. Snyder. Opiate agonists and antagonists discriminated by receptor binding in brain. *Science* 182 (1973): 1359–61.

Schoenenberger, G. A., and M. Monnier. Isolation, partial characterization and activity of a humoral delta-sleep transmitting factor. In *Brain and Sleep*, H. M. Van Praag, ed., pp. 39–69. Amsterdam: H. Meinardi, 1974.

10

L-tryptophan*

It is possible that a hypnotic agent which is not a generalized depressant, but whose action is based on knowledge or at least firm theory about the biochemical basis of sleep, might prove to be an effective hypnotic without serious problems of the sorts mentioned in chapter 8. My laboratory has been investigating the effects of the serotonin precursor l-tryptophan on sleep since 1964. As early as 1965, we suggested that serotonin played a role in the mechanisms underlying sleep (Hartmann, 1965, 1966) and we reported that in some subjects drowsiness and reduced sleep latency were produced by l-tryptophan administration (Hartmann, 1965, 1967). It has since been demonstrated by Jouvet's group (Jouvet and Renalt, 1966; Mouret et al., 1967) and others (Koella et al., 1968; Dement et al., 1972) that serotonin and the serotonergic neurons of the raphe system play a major part in the biochemical mechanisms of sleep. The exact role cannot yet be considered entirely certain; some studies show that when serotonin is maintained at low levels in cats, sleep is eliminated for some days but eventually returns to almost normal levels (although there are qualitative differences; Dement et al., 1972); but clearly serotonin plays a role in the induction or maintenance of normal sleep.

Administration of l-tryptophan has been shown to be an effective way of raising serotonin levels in sites where serotonin naturally occurs in the rat brain (Moir and Eccleston, 1968). In fact, l-tryptophan produces an increase of serotonin specific to serotonin neurons since only these neurons contain tryptophan hydroxylase; administration of 5-OH-tryptophan

* Portions of this chapter are reprinted, with permission, from E. Hartmann, "L-tryptophan as an Hypnotic Agent: A Review" *Waking and Sleeping* 1 (1977): 155–61.

leads to synthesis of serotonin in many other neurons since the decarboxylase enzyme is widespread. Brain serotonin levels may be directly dependent on circulating plasma l-tryptophan levels (Fernstrom and Wurtman, 1971) and these levels respond rapidly to dietary protein and l-tryptophan (Young et al., 1969). Thus, mechanisms are available whereby dietary l-tryptophan or exogenously administered l-tryptophan can have direct effects on brain serotonin and on sleep, although the situation is complicated by many control systems that can alter and regulate l-tryptophan metabolism (Azmitia and McEwen, 1969; Hardeland, 1969; Knox, 1966; Knox et al., 1966).

I shall briefly summarize eleven studies we have completed investigating the effects of l-tryptophan on sleep. The methodology for the studies to be summarized below differed slightly with each individual study; basically, standard methods of human and animal sleep laboratory research were used.

In the rat studies, chronic cortical, hippocampal, and nuchal muscle electrodes were implanted. Each animal had several weeks of adaptation to the laboratory and then had a number of 8-hour recordings following placebo feeding, and one recording after each dose of l-tryptophan—in a balanced sequence.

In the human laboratory studies, the usual electrodes were used to record parietal and occipital EEG, electrooculogram (EOG), and nuchal electromyogram (EMG). All studies were comparisons of l-tryptophan at various doses and placebo under double blind conditions when neither the patient nor the technician running the records or the assistant scoring them knew the identity of the medication. Records were scored according to the usual sleep laboratory criteria (Rechtschaffen and Kales, 1968). Tryptophan and placebo were always administered twenty minutes prior to bedtime. In the studies in which doses of tryptophan of one gram or two grams were employed, tryptophan was administered in 500 mg tablets. In the studies which included larger doses, l-tryptophan in powder form was mixed into applesauce or into a chocolate drink. Placebo consisted of the same vehicle with a few milligrams of quinine or oxaloacetate added to mimic the slightly bitter taste imparted by tryptophan.

In the studies which involved behavioral observation rather than all-night sleep laboratory recordings, a trained observer—in these cases, a doctor or medical student who had no other responsibilities—walked quietly through the ward at 15-minute intervals and noted to the best of his ability whether each patient was awake or asleep. He was permitted to use a category "uncertain" if he could not tell, but this category was almost never used.

All human studies included a subjective report as well as the objective sleep laboratory records or observer ratings. Each morning subjects filled out a form in which they were asked how well they had slept compared to the way they usually sleep on a scale of one to five; how well they felt that morning compared to the way they usually feel on a scale of one to five; there were also questions about side effects, unusual experiences, and dreams.

1. In the rat, we studied the effects of a single administration of doses of 150, 300, 450, and 600 mg/kg of l-tryptophan in a balanced sequence (Hartmann and Chung, 1972a, b). The two higher doses—450 and 600 mg/kg—produced a significant reduction in sleep latency while lower doses produced a trend in the same direction. The overall time spent in synchronized (S) sleep, desynchronized (D) sleep, and waking over 8-hour recording periods was not altered by tryptophan, and no qualitative changes were noted.

2. In a human sleep study employing the usual laboratory recording and scoring procedures, we examined the effects on sleep of l-tryptophan at the doses generally used in tryptophan loading tests—five to ten grams. Each of ten normal subjects was studied for several nights (nonconsecutive) on a single dose in the range of five to ten grams—calculated at approximately 100 mg/kg of body weight, and several nights on placebo. At these doses, l-tryptophan produced a significant

reduction in sleep latency. There was a trend not quite reaching significance toward increased sleep, decreased number of awakenings, and increased D-time (Hartmann, 1967; Hartmann et al., 1971).

3. More recently, we have examined the effects of a wider dose range of l-tryptophan—1 to 15 grams—on human sleep recorded and scored as above. Ten normal males who reported sleep latencies of over 15 minutes at home each slept in the laboratory for an all-night recording on 12 occasions, approximately one night per week. The first two nights were considered adaptation nights and were not used in analysis of the data. On the subsequent ten laboratory nights, each subject took a placebo on three occasions and a dose of l-tryptophan on seven occasions, in a random design. Each dose (1, 2, 3, 4, 5, 10, and 15 grams) was taken once by each subject.

Sleep latency was significantly reduced. The reduction was statistically significant and quite large (50%) even at a dose of one gram (fig. 10.1). Total waking time was also significantly decreased by l-tryptophan. Slow-wave sleep (stages 3 and 4) was unchanged, except that the 10-gram dose produced a significant increase. Desynchronized sleep time (D-time) was significantly decreased when the subjects received the 15-gram dose (Hartmann et al., 1974).

Thus, at doses of one to five grams, l-tryptophan produced a decreased sleep latency and decreased waking without alterations in other aspects of sleep (figs. 10.2, 3).

4. Doses of 2, 3, 4, and 5 grams of l-tryptophan were compared with placebo in a population of 25 hospitalized psychiatric patients complaining of insomnia in addition to their principal psychiatric illness (Hartmann et al., 1971). In this study, each patient was studied for eight nights: four on placebo and one on each of the four doses of l-tryptophan but no EEG recordings were done. Sleep was estimated behaviorally by a trained observer who examined the patients every 15 minutes during the night, using a dim flashlight. The two higher doses of l-tryptophan produced a significant de-

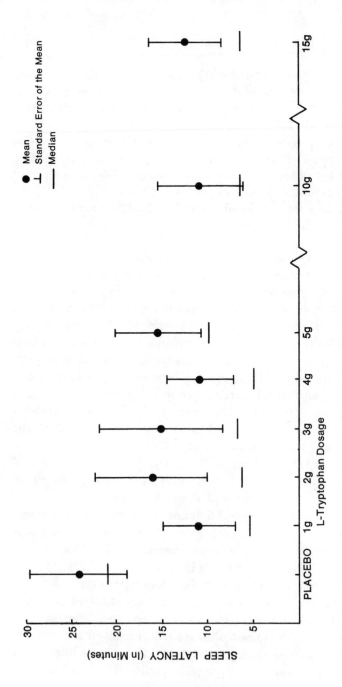

FIGURE 10.1 Sleep Latency after L-Tryptophan

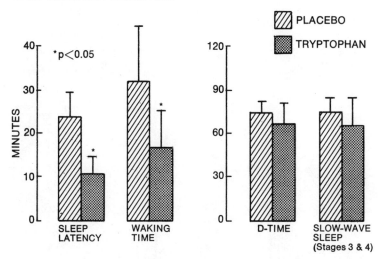

FIGURE 10.2   The Effect on Sleep of L-Tryptophan, 1 gram

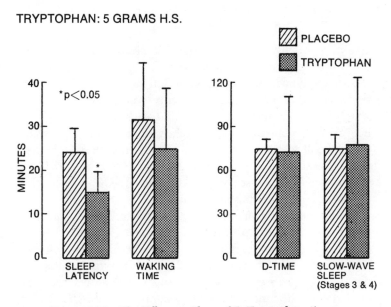

FIGURE 10.3   The Effect on Sleep of L-Tryptophan, 5 grams

ONE NIGHT STUDY

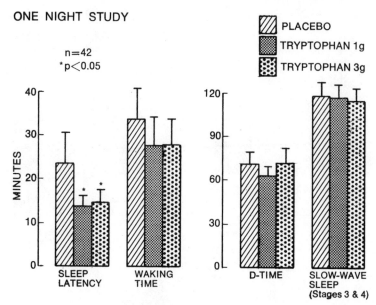

FIGURE 10.4   Effect of L-tryptophan on a Single Night
of Laboratory Sleep

crease in waking time and increase in sleep, while the lower
doses produced nonsignificant trends in the same direction.

5. A study with a design very similar to the above was
performed in a population of twenty women on a geriatric
ward of a mental hospital. We found trends in the same direction as above but no results reached significance. This study
was difficult to interpret because of some data loss and great
intersubject variability, perhaps attributable to a variety of
serious medical illnesses and use of other medications in this
patient group (unpublished study).

6. Another study investigated the effects of five grams of
tryptophan in a group of 29 male chronic alcoholic patients
experiencing insomnia for 2 to 3 weeks following alcohol
withdrawal (Makipour et al., 1972). In this study, tryptophan
significantly decreased sleep latency, significantly increased
total sleep time, and significantly improved subjective sleep
ratings by the patients: we also obtained 24-hour urine levels

of the serotonin metabolite, 5-hydroxy-indoleacetic acid. There was a trend, not reaching significance, toward a positive correlation between reduced sleep latency on tryptophan (tryptophan compared to placebo) and increased 5-hydroxy-indoleacetic acid excretion on tryptophan.

7. A sleep laboratory study was performed on 24 subjects—12 males and 12 females—with mild insomnia, defined as reporting that they required over thirty minutes to fall asleep at home. The subjects slept in the laboratory either once or twice per week. After adaptation, each subject had two nonconsecutive nights on one gram of l-tryptophan and two nights on placebo in a balanced order. One gram of l-tryptophan produced a significant reduction in latency to sleep (stage 1) and in latency to first D-period (Davis et al., 1975).

8. Forty-two normal subjects were studied in the sleep laboratory for one night each. Here the effects of l-tryptophan were investigated on the mild insomnia produced by "sleeping in a strange place" (the strangeness of the place was of course augmented by having electrodes attached to one's head, etc.). Fourteen were given placebo at bedtime, fourteen 1 gram of l-tryptophan, and fourteen 3 grams of l-tryptophan. In this situation, l-tryptophan reduced sleep latency without producing other sleep changes (Elion and Hartmann, 1976; Hartmann and Elion, 1977). The effects of 1 gram and of 3 grams of l-tryptophan were almost identical (fig. 9.4).

9. One long-term study was done on a small number of subjects to investigate whether l-tryptophan produces long-term distortion of normal sleep patterns, as do many hypnotic medications. This study was not designed to investigate sleep latency, so normal, relatively low-latency subjects were used. Four subjects, after five baseline nights, took 1 gram of l-tryptophan nightly and four subjects took 4 grams of l-tryptophan nightly for 28 nights. Each then discontinued tryptophan, and the study continued for 32 more days. Laboratory recordings were made on nights 1–5 and then once per week on tryptophan, and, similarly, nights 1–5, and then once per week during the month after discontinuation. No sleep

stage changes were found which reached significance. The only trend was toward a sustained increase in stage 3 and 4 sleep on tryptophan. Sleep cycling and staging were otherwise unaffected either by long-term tryptophan administration or by discontinuation. As expected, sleep latency tended to be reduced at both doses, but the effect did not reach significance (Hartmann and Cravens, 1975).

10. In one laboratory study, we recently compared the effects on human sleep of several different amino acids. Each of twelve subjects slept in the laboratory for two adaptation nights, and then for eight nonconsecutive experimental nights (once or twice per week). In a balanced order they received each of the following conditions once: l-tryptophan 1 g, l-tryptophan 10 g, glycine 1 g, glycine 10 g, l-leucine 1 g, l-leucine 10 g, placebo powder 1 g, placebo powder 10 g. We found that 10 g of l-tryptophan significantly reduced sleep latency and waking time and 1 g had effects in the same direction, not quite reaching significance. Glycine had no effect on sleep. L-leucine, surprisingly, produced at both doses a trend to reduced sleep latency similar to that found with l-tryptophan 1 g.

11. We also compared the effects of l-tryptophan, l-leucine, and placebo on subjective "sleepiness." Each of thirteen subjects took 4 grams of a powder on three separate evenings one week apart. The powder contained l-tryptophan 4 g, l-leucine 4 g, or placebo, in a balanced order, and was taken at 10 P.M., three hours after the last meal and two to three hours before the subject's usual bedtime. Each subject filled out the Stanford Sleepiness Scale (SSS) before, and every 15 minutes after taking the powders. (The SSS is a simple seven-point scale on which point 1 is "very alert, wide awake" and point 7 is "very sleeply, almost asleep".) Tryptophan produced significantly more "sleepiness" than placebo, starting 30 minutes after administration. The effect was quite dramatic: half of the subjects were either at point 7 or actually asleep two hours after l-tryptophan even though they had not planned to go to

sleep. L-leucine produced a curve part way between placebo and l-tryptophan, but not significantly different from placebo.*

Table 10.1 summarizes the results of these eleven studies. Subjective reports in the laboratory studies showed less change than the objective measures. This is not surprising, since in many of the studies the subjects were normal subjects without sleep complaints. In general, ratings of "How well did you sleep?" showed a nonsignificant trend in the direction of better reported sleep on tryptophan than on placebo, whereas on the question "How well do you feel this morning?" there was no difference whatever between tryptophan and placebo. Reports of side effects were extremely rare. In a few instances, at doses of 5 to 15 grams of l-tryptophan, there were reports of mild nausea at bedtime.

I believe these studies demonstrate that l-tryptophan is effective in reducing sleep latency. This is consistent with the results of Griffiths et al. (1972) who report a reduced waking time after 7.5 grams of l-tryptophan in normal subjects. Also, Wyatt et al. (1970) report a "sedative" effect and an increased sleep time in a group of normal and insomniac subjects, though they report only a nonsignificant reduction in sleep time after l-tryptophan (usually 7.5 grams per day). These studies and others (Griffiths et al., 1972; Oswald et al., 1966; Wyatt et al., 1970) report somewhat conflicting results as to effects of high doses of l-tryptophan on the stages of sleep, but this will not be discussed in detail here. We have also shown that l-tryptophan definitely increases subjective "sleepiness" in normal subjects.

There is general agreement that tryptophan reduces sleep latency and usually reduces waking time; at low doses (1–5 grams) it does so without producing distortions of physio-

* The interesting effects of l-leucine will not be discussed in detail in this chapter. However, the direction of the results is surprising. We had expected that since l-leucine is one of the amino acids which compete with l-tryptophan for transport to the brain, l-leucine might produce less sleepiness or longer sleep latency than placebo. Our findings suggest that other factors are involved—possibly a competition with l-tyrosine (precursor of dopamine and norepinephrine) for transport to the brain.

Table 10.1

Effects of L-tryptophan Compared with Placebo

Study	Type of subjects	Number of subjects (or patients)	Total nights (after adaptation)	Dose of l-tryptophan compared with placebo	Results reaching statistical significance
1	Rats	11	62	150–600 mg/kg	SL reduced at 450, 600 mg/kg
2	NS	10	102	5–10 grams	SL reduced 50%, DT increased slightly
3	MI	10	100	1, 2, 3, 4, 5, 10, 15 grams	SL reduced at 1–15 g, SWS increased at 10 g, DT reduced at 15 g
4	I	24	192[a]	2, 3, 4, 5 grams	SL reduced, ST increased (4, 5 g)
5	I-G	20	160[a]	5 grams	No significant effect
6	I	29	126[a]	5 grams	SL reduced, ST increased, SQS improved
7	MI	24	96	1 gram	SL reduced, DL reduced
8	NS	42	42	1, 3 grams	SL reduced, equally by 1 and 3 grams
9	NS	8	128	1, 4 grams	No long-term changes, No changes on discontinuation
10	MI	12	96	1, 10 grams	SL, waking time decreased (10 g dose)
11	NS	13	—	4 grams	"Sleepiness" increased

DL = D-latency; DT = D-time; G = geriatric population; I = insomniacs; MI = mild insomniacs (long-latency subjects); NS = normal human subjects; SL = sleep latency; SQS= subjective quality of sleep; ST = sleep time; SWS = slow-wave sleep.
[a] Behavioral observation; no laboratory recordings.

logical sleep as measured by EEG recordings. Therefore, it avoids at least one of the major problems of hypnotic medication listed in chapter 7. Complete data are not available to determine whether it would be a useful hypnotic in other senses, but I would suggest at least the following probable advantages.

Certainly, l-tryptophan should be one of the safer drugs available, since 1 to 2 grams are ingested daily in the normal diet. However, an amino acid administered in pure form can produce very different effects from the same amount in a mixture of amino acids and other food substances. Investigations of toxicity after short- and long-term administration of l-tryptophan is obviously indicated. Problems of allergy or idiosyncrasy should be nonexistent or extremely rare, and have not been reported as yet. Long-term use of high doses of l-tryptophan could have certain potential dangers: a highly abnormal mixture of amino acids could reduce or alter protein synthesis; this could represent a danger, especially in the growing organism. Also, it has been reported that implantation of crystals of certain tryptophan metabolites into the bladder was carcinogenic in animals (Bryan, 1971). This will require further investigation. However, l-tryptophan is already in use on a long-term basis as an antidepressant in Great Britain: doses of 6 to 9 grams per day have been taken for a period of many months by several thousand patients with reports of very few side effects, and no serious side effects (A. Coppen, personal communication). In our two hundred subjects and patients, we had no side effects other than a few reports of nausea at the higher doses of l-tryptophan. In no study were significantly more side effects found after l-tryptophan than after placebo.

The question of tryptophan as a drug of abuse has not yet arisen. However, sleep EEG changes were found neither on long-term administration nor during the month after withdrawal, nor were any psychological symptoms reported during these periods by normal subjects in our studies; and no problems on withdrawal have been reported in Great Britain.

This leads one to hope that addiction and withdrawal problems would be minimal or absent with l-tryptophan.

L-tryptophan is rapidly metabolized and cleared by the body, since it is ingested every day and all the necessary enzymes are already present in active form. Indeed, our sleep recordings show that the effects on sleep EEGs seem to last only a few hours: sleep latency is almost always shortened in our studies, and waking time is significantly reduced in the early portions of the night. Waking time in the last hours of sleep is not altered. This leads to the hope that tolerance to tryptophan would not be built up by the body on a long-term basis.

It is of interest that in study 3 there was a flat dose response curve for sleep latency: the full effect was produced by 1 gram and there was no increase on higher doses. Similarly, in study 8 1 gram and 3 grams of l-tryptophan produced indistinguishable results. There may be a transport system, or perhaps an enzyme system, that is saturated in normal subjects by administration of 1 gram of l-tryptophan, at least during the initial period when sleep onset would be affected. In clinical terms, this suggests that if tryptophan is to be used to reduce sleep latency, 1 gram may be a sufficient dose.

The investigations summarized here have, I believe, demonstrated the efficacy of l-tryptophan in reducing sleep latency and waking time, as well as increasing subjective "sleepiness" in the subjects and patients studied. They have not been directed to determining the mechanism of action. The increase in brain serotonin, already discussed, would appear most likely to be involved. An alternate or contributory mechanism could be interference with dopamine or norepinephrine synthesis by competion with tyrosine or DOPA; and even more indirect mechanisms of action cannot be entirely ruled out.

In addition to the specific studies detailed above, involving a total of 193 subjects and patients, I have prescribed l-tryptophan to about 35 patients on clinical grounds. The dosage used was 1–5 grams. The patients have not been followed up in a systematic fashion, but a number have definitely benefited from treatment, and none has reported disturbing side effects. My impression from these studies and clinical trials is that l-tryptophan can be especially useful in sleep-onset insomnia. The patients described the effects as an increase in normal tiredness—they were seldom "knocked out": thus l-tryptophan, as might be expected, is apparently not a powerful CNS depressant and would presumably not be useful for a severely agitated insomniac patient.

Summary

Eleven studies have been reported on which, along with data from other laboratories, support and confirm the sleep-inducing properties of the amino acid l-tryptophan. L-tryptophan reduces sleep latency (time taken to fall asleep) in rats, in normal humans, and in mild insomniacs at a dose as low as 1 gram. This is of importance, since l-tryptophan is a constituent of protein and 0.5 to 2.0 grams are ingested in the normal daily diet; thus, l-tryptophan can be thought of as a natural food substance rather than as a drug. At a single dose of up to 5 grams it does not distort normal sleep stage patterns; nor is sleep distorted by long-term administration. Studies of l-tryptophan in clinical insomniac populations are in progress, but the results are not yet available, and studies of safety are needed; but it appears quite possible that l-tryptophan will turn out to be a safe and useful sleeping pill. Its probable mechanism of action involves an increase of brain serotonin in brain serotoninergic neurons; thus, its action is related to the known chemistry of sleep and it is not a general central nervous system depressant.

Considering the three approaches to the development of a safe and rational sleeping pill, it appears that l-tryptophan offers the greatest clinical potential in the near future. The other two approaches (chap. 9), could perhaps lead to rational sleeping medication in the more distant future.

References

Azmitia, E. C., Jr., and B. S. McEwen. Corticosterone regulation of tryptophane hydroxylase in midbrain of the rat. *Science* 155 (1969): 1274–76.

Bryan, G. T. The role of urinary tryptophan metabolites in the etiology of bladder cancer. *Am. J. Clin. Nutrition* 24 (1971): 841–47.

Coppen, Alec. Personal communications to the author. Also personal communications from Cambrian Chemicals Ltd. and from the Medicines Council of Great Britain.

Davis, D.; J. Tyler; and E. Hartmann. Effects on human sleep of l-tryptophane, 1 and 2 grams. In *Sleep Research*, 4:72. Los Angeles, Brain Information Service, UCLA, 1975.

Dement, W. C.; M. M. Mitler; and S. J. Henriksen. Sleep changes during chronic administration of parachlorophenylalamine. *Rev. Can. Biol.* 31 (Suppl.) (1972): 239–46.

Elion, R., and E. Hartmann. The effects of l-tryptophane on the first night of sleep. *Sleep Research*, 5:55, 1976.

Fernstrom, J. D., and R. J. Wurtmann. Brain serotonin content: Physiological dependence on plasma tryptophan levels. *Science* 173 (1971): 149–52.

Griffiths, W. J.; B. K. Lester; J. D. Couiter; and H. L. Williams. Tryptophan and sleep in young adults. *Psychophysiology* 9 (1972): 345–46.

Hardeland, R. Circadian rhythmicity and regulation of enzymes of tryptophane metabolism in rat liver and kidney. *Z. Vergl. Physiologie* 63 (1969): 119.

Hartmann, E. Serotonin and dreaming. Report to the Association for the Psychophysiological Study of Sleep. Washington, D.C., March 1965.

———. Some studies on the biochemistry of dreaming sleep. Proceedings of the IV World Congress of Psychiatry. Madrid, September 1966. *Excerpta Medica Int. Cong. Series* 150 (1966): 3100–02.

———. The effect of tryptophane on the sleep-dream cycle in man. *Psychonom.* 8 (1967): 479–80.

Hartmann, E.; R. Chung; and C. P. Chien. L-tryptophane and sleep. *Psychopharmacologia* 19 (1971): 114–27.

Hartmann, E.; and R. Chung. L-tryptophane: Effect on sleep in the normal rat and the rat with lowered brain catecholamines. *Psychophysiology* 9 (1972a): 87–88.

————. Sleep-inducing effects of l-tryptophane. *J. Pharm. Pharmacol.* 24 (1972): 252–53.

Hartmann, E.; J. Cravens; and S. List. Hypnotic effects of l-tryptophane. *Arch. Gen. Psychiat.* 31 (1974): 394–97.

Hartmann, E., and J. Cravens. Effects of long-term administration of l-tryptophane on human sleep. *Sleep Research,* 4:76. Los Angeles, Brain Information Service, UCLA, 1975.

Hartmann, E., and R. Elion. The insomnia of "sleeping in a strange place": effects of l-tryptophan. *Psychopharmacology* 53 (1977): 131–33.

Jouvet, M., and J. Renalt. Insomnie persistante après lesions des noyaux du raphe chez le chat. *C. R. Soc. Biol.* 160 (1966): 1461–. 65.

Kagen, F.; T. Harwood; K. Rickels; A. D. Rudzik; and H. Sorer. Hypnotics: Methods of Development and Evaluation. New York: Spectrum Publications, 1974.

Kales, A.; R. O. Bixler; T.-L. Tan; M. B. Scharf; and J. D. Kales. Chronic hypnotic-drug use ineffectiveness, drug-withdrawal insomnia, and dependence. *JAMA* 227 (1974): 513–17.

Knox, W. E. The regulation of tryptophane pyrrolase activity by tryptophane. *Adv. Enzyme Regul.* 4 (1966): 287–97.

Knox, W. E.; M. M. Piras; and K. Tokuyama. Induction of tryptophane pyrrolase in rat liver by physiological amounts of hydrocortisone and secreted glucocorticoids. *Enzyme Biol. Clin.* 7 (1966): 1–10.

Koella, W. P.; A. Feldstein; and J. Czicman. The effect of parachlorphenylalamine on the sleep of cats. *Electroenceph. Clin. Neurophysiol.* 25 (1968): 481.

Makipour, H.; F. L. Iber; and E. Hartmann. Effects of l-tryptophane on sleep in hospitalized insomniac patients. Reports to the Association for the Psychophysiological Study of Sleep, Lake Minnewaska, New York, 1972. Abstract. *Sleep Research,* Los Angeles Brain Information Service, UCLA, 1972.

Moir, A. T. B., and D. Eccleston. The effects of precursor loading in the cerebral metabolism of 5-hydroxyindoles. *J. Neurochem.* 15 (1968): 1093–1108.

Mourct, J.; P. Bobillier; and M. Jouvet. Effets de la parachlorophenylalamine sur le sommeil du rat. *C. R. Soc. Biol.* 161 (1967): 1600–03.

Oswald, I.; G. W. Ashcroft; R. J. Berger; D. Eccleston; J. L.

Evans; and V. R. Thacore. Some experiments in the chemistry of normal sleep. *Br. J. Psychiatry* 112 (1966): 391–99.

Rechtschaffen, A., and A. Kales. A manual of standardized terminology techniques and scoring systems for sleep stages of human subjects. Public Health Service, Washington D.C.: U.S. Government Printing Office, 1968.

Wyatt, R. J.; D. J. Kupfer; A. Sjoerdsma; et al. Effects of l-tryptophane (a natural sedative) on human sleep. *Lancet,* October 24, 1970, pp. 842–45.

Young, V. R.; M. A. Hussein; E. Murray; N. S. Schrimshaw. Tryptophane intake, spacing of meals, and diurnal fluctuations of plasma tryptophane in man. *Am. J. Clin. Nutr.* 22 (1969): 1563–67.

11

The Sleeping Pill: Conclusions

The sleeping pill in some form has been part of medicine and of human interaction for centuries and will probably continue in these roles, though perhaps to a diminished extent.

Sleeping pills are presumably used to treat insomnia. However, it is essential to remember that insomnia is not an illness for which a sleeping pill is the cure. Insomnia is a symptom or final common path resulting from many underlying causes. Among these are serious depression, several kinds of anxiety, and numerous medical diseases, including a number of sleep-related conditions as well as various sources of pain and discomfort. Some of these, of course, have other causes in their turn.

Whenever possible, treatment for insomnia should be treatment for a specific illness or underlying cause. Thus, it will sometimes include simply psychological support, a change in life patterns, or a change in environment; it will at other times involve psychotherapy. Sometimes treatment will be aimed at a specific medical condition that caused pain and discomfort. Some cases of insomnia secondary to sleep apnea will require surgical treatment (tracheotomy). Overall, in a great many instances insomnia is best treated without medication. When medication is required, it will frequently be an antidepressant, antipsychotic, or other medication intended to treat specific underlying conditions, rather than a sleeping pill aimed simply at the symptom of inability to sleep.

Yet there are times when a sleeping pill is appropriate: these include temporary situational insomnias in which it is understood by both patient and doctor that medication is being used for a short time. Periods of sleep difficulty associated with surgery or other clearly defined medical conditions are also good reasons for short-term use of sleeping pills. Included may be certain long-term insomnias that cannot as yet be related to a specific underlying cause, or which are related to an underlying cause with no known treatment, and perhaps certain rare neurological problems involving actual neurological or chemical sleep mechanisms in the brain.

Sleeping pills are presently overprescribed and overused. I have examined some of the practical and psychological reasons for this. As sleeping pills are being used now, my conclusion is that the overall risks outweigh the overall benefits. If a drug is used only for very specific indications, if the drug to be used is carefully chosen, and if new drugs are developed that relate specifically to the biology and chemistry of sleep, this low benefit-to-risk ratio will no longer apply.

Currently prescribed hypnotics are mostly nonspecific CNS depressants whose mode of action has nothing to do with the normal biology of sleep. I have examined the dangers in their use, including accidental death. (This danger increases for persons who have specific sleep pathologies or are taking other medication.) A group of newer hypnotics—the benzodiazepines—have a definite advantage in terms of safety. Side effects do occur, but there is little respiratory depression, so that deaths are rare. Yet in other ways these drugs are also general depressants and their mechanism of action is not known. I have also discussed some possible alternative sleeping medications based on increasing knowledge of the biochemistry of sleep. I have suggested three possibly useful lines of investigation: substances related to the short-chain brain peptides; substances that would reduce brain dopamine activity; and l-tryptophan or related substances which increase levels or activity of brain serotonin.

The many possible psychological as well as medical reasons for taking sleeping pills have been discussed. It has been pointed out that many of these are poor reasons for risking the multiple possible harmful effects of these medications. Yet symbolic psychological factors are powerful and will not suddenly vanish when exposed to the light of reason.

I believe that progress must and will take place along two paths: safer, more rational, and probably more natural substances (perhaps including l-tryptophan) will be used increasingly; and I hope that the overall use of sleeping pills will gradually decrease as we understand and accept the ways in which sleeping pills have been misused and the alternatives to their use. Considering the recent history of mankind—the breathtakingly rapid forward sprints in technology and the uncertain, slow meanderings elsewhere—I think the first path will turn out to be the easier one. In other words, I believe that the use of new and more rational sleeping pills will precede our ability to adjust our adaptive mechanisms in such a way as greatly to reduce the need for sleeping pills, though eventually the latter will also occur.

Appendix A

The Effects of
Drugs on Sleep:
Laboratory Studies

The following five studies from my laboratory investigate the long-term effects of drug administration upon laboratory-recorded sleep. These can be considered basic pharmacological studies in which we observed short-term effects, long-term effects, and effects after discontinuation, of a group of important drugs upon laboratory-recorded sleep as well as subjects' impressions of sleep, from a group of carefully chosen, reliable normal subjects.

In terms of the historical development of sleep pharmacology, these studies are relatively recent and relatively sophisticated. A series of previous studies in many laboratories had demonstrated effects on sleep of a single night of drug administration; had discovered that the first night of laboratory sleep is somewhat unusual, so that "adaptation" is required; and had shown that different and unexpected effects sometimes occur when a drug is administered over a period of days, and when it is withdrawn. These paved the way for, and in a sense created the necessity for, long-term studies like the ones presented here.

Since these are basic pharmacological studies we did not use insomniacs, and therefore these cannot be considered direct studies of the efficacy of sleeping medications for the improvement of sleep in insomniacs. These long-term studies will demonstrate the methodology of laboratory sleep studies, as well as providing some important specific results.

Five "drugs" are studied in detail. The first is placebo; we consider it very important to study effects of short- and long-term placebo administration for comparisons with effects of other medications. This provides a necessary control for studies of the other drugs. The other medications studied include amitriptyline, now the most widely used antidepressant medication which is also used frequently in treating insomnia, especially in middle-aged persons who are suspected of being depressed (see chap. 5). Chlorpromazine is studied as the major antipsychotic drug; it is a dopamine receptor blocker and, as we have seen, there are reasons why this might make it an effective hypnotic medication. At present, chlorpromazine is not generally used as a hypnotic, except in patients also taking it as an antipsychotic agent; but it does clearly have hypnotic properties. Chloral hydrate is one of the oldest and clinically most widely used of the presently available hypnotic agents. We also studied one of the benzodiazepenes—chlordiazepoxide (Librium): Although at present chlordiazepoxide and diazepam (Valium) are used more commonly in the daytime as "tranquilizers," while flurazepam (Dalmane) is used more at night as a hypnotic, it is clear from sleep and other studies that the three have extremely similar properties. Chlordiazepoxide was the most widely used member of the group at the time these studies were initiated.

Our original studies also included reserpine, a drug of great theoretical importance used as an antihypertensive and an antipsychotic; however, since reserpine is not used in any way as a sleeping medication, that study is not reproduced here. In all cases, various preliminary short-term studies were done to establish, for each medication, one dose that would be in the clinical range and yet could be tolerated by normal subjects on long-term administration. Thus, in the present studies, only one dose of each medication is investigated and compared with placebo.

The Effects of Long-Term Administration of Psychotropic Drugs on Human Sleep: Methodology and the Effects of Placebo

Ernest Hartmann and James Cravens

Sleep and Dream Laboratory, Boston State Hospital
Department of Psychiatry, Tufts University School of Medicine

Abstract. These papers present the effects on human sleep of long-term administration of reserpine (0.50 mg/day), amitriptyline (50 mg/day), chlorpromazine (50 mg/day), chloral hydrate (500 mg/day), chlordiazepoxide (50 mg/day), and placebo.

This initial paper describes in detail the methodology of the entire study, which involves six 60-day drug periods for each subject completing the protocol—one period on each of the five drugs and one period on placebo, in a balanced design. Measures of laboratory sleep, home sleep, and mood were obtained throughout the study.

Comparisons between the long placebo-only period of this study and the more usual "baseline" period—laboratory nights 4–6—revealed a significantly higher total desynchronized sleep time (D-time) and D-time percent in the placebo period. Other variables were not significantly different. Some clear changes over time within the long placebo period are also described.

We report here on the effects on normal human subjects of the daily administration for 28 days of six medications—reserpine, amitriptyline, chlorpromazine, chloral hydrate, chlordiazepoxide, and placebo. Effects on laboratory sleep, home sleep, and mood were studied. In this initial paper we present our methodology in detail and discuss other recent methodologies used for drug studies in the sleep laboratory; we then present results on the effects of placebo administration.

Since the inception of modern sleep research in the middle 1950's, there have been a large number of studies of drug effects on sleep, some of which will be reviewed in detail later. By and large, these studies have confirmed that all-night EEG and polygraphic recordings may provide a number of replicable measures of central nervous system activity, and that these measures are often sensitive to the effects of drugs at relatively low dosages in the clinical range, which may produce no discernible effects on behavior or subjective state.

Because of the great expense involved in laboratory sleep studies, almost all investigations to date have involved administration of medication for one night or for several nights to a small number of subjects. Such designs of course do not allow for investigation of any long-term effect, investigation of the gradual adaptation (tolerance) or lack of adaptation of various sleep measures to the medication, nor for the study of the clinically very important period after discontinuation of medication, a time when effects are sometimes especially pronounced.

Furthermore, it has been found, not surprisingly, that adaptation to the sleep laboratory sometimes takes several nights, or even longer (Agnew, Webb, and Williams, 1967; Hartmann, 1967). The simple fact that the subject is sleeping in an unfamiliar and somewhat unusual setting, with wires pasted to his head, and the knowledge that an experimenter is nearby monitoring his sleep, can hardly help having an effect on the subject's sleep. Although sleep researchers have been aware of this fact, they have dealt with it in the usual short-term studies only by allowing one, or occasionally two or three nights of adaptation, and then whenever possible balancing drug and placebo nights. Often drug nights can be compared only to preceding "baseline" nights. The present long-term study design not only allows a longer adaptation and baseline period than usual, but by introducing an entire two-month period of study on placebo, taken in exactly the same way as other medications, allows a comparison of placebo with early baseline nights, and also allows each drug to be compared to the effects of placebo given in an identical protocol in the same subjects.

In addition, some medications may have very different effects on long-term administration (the way they are usually taken), as opposed to the first day of administration. As one example, some of the antidepressants, especially amitriptyline, studied here, are known to produce drowsiness on the first day of administration but have little antidepressant effect until after about two weeks of continuous administration. We have shown that amitriptyline has a dramatic effect on sleep when first administered (Hartmann, 1968a; 1968b), but this could be completely unrelated to the antidepressant effect; the present study will allow us to look at the changes after weeks of continuous administration to find possible relationships with the clinical action. Moreover, some drugs such as chloral hydrate may lose their effectiveness as hypnotics upon continuous administration (Kales, Kales, Scharf, and Tan, 1970). The present study was designed to overcome most of these problems by studying all drugs over a long period of time (one month of administration) followed by an equally long study time after discontinuation of medication. This of course involved a large number of nights of study; we believe nonetheless that this design is relatively economic and that we achieved a number of objectives with the minimum number of nights necessary (see below).

METHOD

Subjects   In a study such as this, where each subject takes part for 12–18 months, and a great deal of time, effort, and money is expended upon each, subject selection becomes a very important procedure. Subjects were selected from a group of normal, healthy young males, 21–35 years of age. Females were not used because of possible changes in the sleep patterns (Hartmann, 1966) and in drug effects with the menstrual cycle. Since sleep patterns of course vary with age, we studied a fairly narrow range of ages.

Volunteers were first obtained by placing a classified advertisement in several newspapers on three occasions over a period of three years. The number of telephone inquiries was always large, but a short conversation immediately eliminated about 40% of the callers on the basis of health, sleep habits, or unwillingness to participate once they were made aware of the long-term nature of the study.

To those applicants who passed this "telephone screening" we sent a set of forms: A sleep questionnaire; the Cornell Index (Brodman, Erdman, Lorge, Wolff, and Broadbent, 1949); Rotter Incomplete Sentences Form (Rotter and Willerman, 1947); and a sleep log to be filled out daily for two weeks. Of the approximately 200 sets of forms sent out over three years, only about half were returned. This was expected and intended, since most of those who lacked the interest or motivation to fill out these forms more than likely would have lacked interest and motivation enough to complete this lengthy study. The forms themselves allowed us a more complex screening for regularity of life style and sleep patterns, and gave us some measures of physical and psychological health.

Finally about 35 applicants were asked to come to the laboratory for more extensive interviews and an MMPI. Applicants were rejected if they were suffering from any serious medical or psychiatric illness, if they were taking medication, except for small quantities of nicotine, alcohol, cannabis, or caffeine, or if they scored more than two standard deviations above the mean on any of the clinical scales on the MMPI except Mf (masculine-feminine). Applicants were also rejected if their sleep was very irregular, if they frequently took naps, if their lives seemed likely to change greatly within the next year, or if they seemed unable to appreciate the difficulties and inconveniences of such a long study involving prolonged medication periods.

Laboratory and
Home Schedule   Each subject chosen was first studied for three laboratory nights at approximately one-week

intervals which were considered adaptation nights. As this point, it was still possible for us to eliminate a subject from further study if for some reason he found the laboratory especially disturbing, or if his sleep records had some characteristics that might make them very difficult for us to score later. Each accepted subject then slept in the laboratory for three further nights at approximately one-week intervals (nights 4–6), which will be referred to as baseline nights. We shall discuss these later in relation to the differences between the later placebo period and the baseline nights. In presenting the results of the drug studies, however, the baseline period will not be considered; rather, each two-month drug period is compared to the two-month placebo period (see below), not the baseline period, in the same subject.

Each subject then started on a protocol which involved six 60-day study periods, one for each medication condition. Each 60-day study period involved a single medication and the order of the medications was determined by a 6×6 Latin square design balanced for drug order. Fourteen subjects completed enough of it to make their data useable (2 months or more) and eight subjects completed the entire 12–18 months of study.

In each 60-day study period subjects took medication (one pink or red capsule) 20 min before bedtime on 28 consecutive nights. They each slept in the laboratory the first five nights on medication and then once per week for the remaining time on medication. Then medication was discontinued for at least 32 days before the beginning of the next study period; the subject slept in the laboratory the first six nights after discontinuation of medication and one night per week for the remainder of the time off medication (Fig. 1). The first five nights *on* medication and the first six nights *off* medication were always laboratory nights. There was some flexibility in the timing of the subsequent one-per-week nights. Insofar as possible, weekend nights were avoided since even the most regular sleepers are likely to vary their sleep patterns on weekends. The first nights *on* and *off* medication were usually

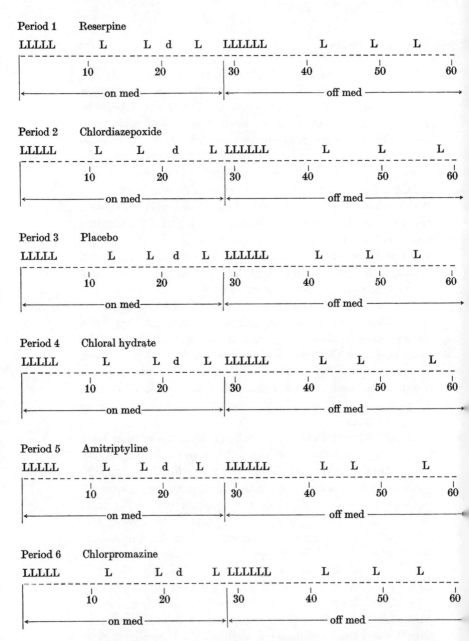

Fig. 1. Typical schedule for a subject on long-term drug study. The six 60-day periods are preceded by an adaptation and baseline period (see text). A home log is filled out every morning, days 1–60 on each study; POMS, every 7th day. ...oratory sleep nights are indicated by an L; d indicates subject awakened for ...m reports.

Monday nights. An attempt was made to be aware of each subject's life style, habits, and plans to assure his cooperation in scheduling laboratory sleep nights and to ensure that the laboratory nights were as "normal" as possible. Studies were planned so that any expected disruptions or irregular events in the subjects' lives (exams, vacations, crucial projects at work) would fall between two study periods (i.e., *after* the 32 days of off-medication study but before the next medication period).

Around the eighteenth night of each study period an additional laboratory sleep night was scheduled during which subjects were awakened from D-periods (desynchronized or REM sleep periods) for dream recall—about 5 min into the first and 10 min into the remaining D-periods. On these recall nights, awakenings were made and questions asked by a technician who was blind as to drug condition. The same technician ran every dream recall night throughout the study. After awakening the subject and asking him what had been going through his mind the technician chose from a standard list the questions he felt were needed to elaborate on the content the subject had initially given. The recall night was scheduled so as always to precede the next regular laboratory night by at least four nights to insure that subjects had recovered from the slight amount of D-deprivation incurred by the awakenings.

At some time during the third or fourth week on medication subjects were interviewed by an investigator (EH) blind as to drug condition, regarding drug effects, any important events in the subjects' lives, etc. These interviews were also used to maintain rapport with the subject and to obtain advance warning of any difficult life situations that might arise during the extremely long study period required.

Each morning of the entire study period subjects filled out home sleep logs regarding sleep times, quality of sleep, events of previous day, dreams recalled, any naps, and any unusual psychological or physiological events (Table 1). Each Sunday morning the subjects filled out an adjective check list (the

TABLE 1.

Questions answered daily in the home log

For each night of sleep

Day and Date (evening)

Questions 1–3 refer to day before sleep period (date above).

1. Any naps? alcohol? medication of any kind (except for this study)?
   If yes, please describe.
2. Any unusual activities or occurrences that might have influenced your
   sleep (e.g., physical exercise, sexual intercourse, upsetting news,
   exams, major changes in daily routine, etc.)?
3. Time to bed?
4. Time you got up this morning?
5. How much sleep do you think you had?
   For questions 6 and 7 use following rating system:
   5 = much better
   4 = a little better
   3 = same as usual
   2 = a little worse
   1 = much worse than usual
6. How well did you sleep compared to the way you usually sleep?
7. How do you feel this morning?
8. Any dreams? If yes, please describe briefly, including mood in dream
   and any unusual features.
9. Do you feel sick in any way whatever?
   Any unusual physical feelings? If yes, please describe.
10. Any unusual psychological feelings this morning or during the past
    day? More or less depressed, anxious, or angry than usual? If yes,
    please describe.
11. If you answered yes to questions 9 or 10, do you think that it may
    be due to the medicine you are taking or is it explainable in other
    ways?

POMS [McNair, Lorr, and Droppleman, 1971]) describing
their mood state for the previous week.

Subjects were paid $10 per laboratory night for participa-
tion in the study so that each subject who completed the
protocol earned about $1100. Seven dollars per night was paid
immediately, while the other $3 per night was retained to be
paid only at the end of the study to provide additional motivation for completion.

Medications studied were reserpine 0.50 mg per day, amitriptyline 50 mg per day, chlorpromazine 50 mg per day,
chloral hydrate 500 mg per day, and chlordiazepoxide 50 mg
per day, in addition to placebo.

Recording and Scoring   The sleep laboratory is equipped with three quiet, comfortable (air-conditioned, sound-at-tentuated) sleep rooms. The EEG machines used are a Grass Model IV (8 channels) and a Grass model VI 8–2 (10 channels). The four usual channels for sleep recording were used (Rechtschaffen and Kales, 1968): one EEG (parietal lead referred to common reference (typically C_4 versus A_1); two EOGs (outer canthus of each eye referred to common reference, E_1 versus $A_1 + E_2$ versus A_1); one EMG (bipolar, chin versus chin); and one additional EEG (occipital to common reference, O_2 versus A_1). By attaching a few extra electrodes (total of nine in all), it was usually possible to obtain good recordings, even if one or two electrodes became lost during the night, without waking subjects to reapply electrodes. Electrodes were 72″ Grass silver cup electrodes, filled with Cambridge Electrode Jelly, with scalp electrodes secured with gauze and collodion and other electrodes secured with Johnson & Johnson Surgical Tape.

Technicians were all young males and the number of active technicians was never larger than three so that subjects coming into the laboratory to sleep usually encountered a familiar situation. Technicians were instructed to make notes on any unusual circumstances or events which may in any way have had an effect on the subjects' sleep.

Scoring of the sleep records was done by scorers trained in our laboratory to score sleep records according to the Rechtschaffen and Kales recommendations (1968). Records were scored for waking, descending stage 1, stage 2, stage 3, stage 4, D-state, and body movements. Records for each subject were scored blind by a single scorer in random order and every tenth record was scored by another individual scorer as well. Periodic scoring meetings were held to help keep scoring standardized for the laboratory. Whenever possible the last laboratory night off medication (approximately night 56) was scored immediately to make sure it was close to the subject's baseline on major sleep parameters. It was planned to postpone the next study period if this last night showed unusual effects that could be related to long-term drug withdrawal, but this did not occur. Finally, score sheets for each night were keypunched for computer analysis and the following laboratory sleep variables were calculated: time spent in each stage of sleep, total sleep time, time in each stage as a percent of total sleep, waking time, number of awakenings, number of body movements, number of D-periods, sleep latency, D-latency, stage 4 latency, total slow-wave sleep time, cycle length, number of stage shifts, and disturbance index.[1] For each laboratory sleep night these variables were tabulated for the entire record, the first 3 h of record, the second 3 h of record, the first 6 h of record, and the first 6 h of sleep. Data from home logs and POMS mood forms was coded and similarly tabulated by computer.

Several simple statistical measures were applied to the data: The drug effects were analyzed first of all by *t*-tests for correlated samples across certain intervals chosen to be of interest, *i.e.*, effects of drug for the first night on medication, first three nights on and first five nights on, remaining nights on, all nights on, last night on, first night off, second night off, third night off, first three nights off, second three nights off, first six nights off, remaining nights off, last night off, and all nights off.

Also, correlation coefficients (for the entire night as well as for the first 6 h) were obtained between all laboratory variables, between all the home variables, and between these two groups of variables. These correlations were calculated overall, and separately on placebo and on each drug condition to enable us to examine drug effects on these correlations.

---

1. D-periods: number of occurrences of D-sleep separated from other occurrences of D-sleep by more than 15 min.

Sleep latency: time spent from beginning of record until first stage 1 which leads to stage 2.

D-latency: total time *asleep* before initial D-period.

Stage 4-latency: total time asleep before first occurrence of stage 4.

Total Slow-wave sleep: sum of times spent in stage 3 and stage 4.

Cycle length: average time between ends of D-periods.

Disturbance Index: sum of body movements and (30 sec) pages of waking.

Multiple Regression analyses were performed in certain instances to answer questions of specific interest, i.e., what combination of laboratory variables best "accounts for" the variance in subjective estimates of good sleep, etc. Certain more complex comparisons were performed as well and will be discussed in the appropriate places in subsequent papers.

Comparison of Different Designs   There are, of course, different methodologies that could have been used in a study of this kind. One reasonable alternative to our present design, and an alternative that has frequently been used (Kales, Preston, Tan, and Allen, 1970; Kales, Malmstrom, Kee, Kales, and Tan, 1969) is the use of separate subjects for each drug study—thus involving a much larger group of subjects for the total study. Such a design has the advantage of avoiding any possible contaminating effects of a drug upon subsequent drug periods— a possibility we believe caused minimal disturbance here because of the long time intervals, but which cannot be completely disregarded even with the 32–50 days which intervened between drug periods in our design. (Also, the design of this study allowed us to test whether important parameters had returned to baseline, since we attempted to score immediately the last night off medication and postpone the next drug study if there was any question of an unusual night at this time.) The design involving many separate subjects may also have certain statistical advantages (Lana and Lubin, 1963). However, in our opinion these advantages were balanced or outweighed by certain others: for one thing, we feel much more comfortable working with the same carefully screened subjects over a long period of time; we are able to get to know them better through a series of spaced interviews, etc. Likewise, a subject gets to know the laboratory and personnel; perhaps most important is that with familiarity with the laboratory routine and its rationale, the subject tends to become increasingly cooperative and reliable; to the best of our knowledge, there was very little "cheating" on medications or naps, and there were almost no missed nights. Furthermore, the subject's knowledge that he will be in the laboratory study for a period of 1 to 2 years serves as a selective factor, selecting subjects who are reliable and willing to participate in the various phases of the experiments such as filling out numerous forms, etc.[2] Moreover, our design allows us to study effects of long-term administration of placebo compared to a subject's own baseline: a comparison which could not be made using the other design. Similarly, our crossover design allows a comparison of different drugs with one another, as well as with placebo, in a matched (identical) sample. For instance, in this series one may study the possible hypnotic effects of chlorpromazine, chlordiazepoxide, or amitriptyline by comparing sleep latency, waking time, etc. on these drugs directly with sleep latency or waking time on chloral hydrate, as well as on placebo, in the same subjects.

Finally, there is the question of number of nights that must be run to obtain a given result: the results of this study demonstrate what we suspected before, that merely comparing a drug period to a prior baseline does not give an entirely accurate measure of drug versus placebo effects. For a long-term study one should rather compare a drug period with an identical period on placebo. (For instance, with chloral hydrate we found that D-time clearly rose several days after drug discontinuation (Hartmann and Cravens, 1973) and this was a significant increase for the entire group relative to baseline. However, it turned out that the curve on placebo had an almost identical rise several days after discontinuation—see below—so that clearly this was not a drug effect.) Therefore in the alternative design (subjects studied for one drug each) each subject should have an entire drug period and an entire placebo period. Such a design, however, would require five subjects each taking part in two 60-day study periods, or in other words, 20 months of sleep study, to

2. Psychologically this could lead to a sample skewed toward obsessive compulsive persons, but our subjects showed little evidence of this.

obtain approximately the information which we obtained in one subject studied for six 60-day periods, including a placebo period, for a total of 12 months of sleep study. Considering the amount of difficulty and labor involved in obtaining and scoring a single night of sleep, this saving is not inconsiderable.

Ideally, of course, a large long-term drug study such as this should also have investigated the effects of several dosages of each drug to obtain a dose-response curve. We have performed some dose-response studies of single night effects (Hartmann, 1968a; 1968b; Hartmann, Cravens, and List, 1973). However, our preliminary studies, and a search through other studies, published and unpublished, in which the drugs of interest to us had been administered over longer periods of time to normal subjects, indicated somewhat to our surprise that no meaningful dose-response study was possible for long-term administration of these drugs to normal human subjects. As an example, in the case of chlorpromazine, the dose we finally chose for long-term study was 50 mg per day. This is certainly towards the lower end of the clinical range and the interest in a dose-response curve would be especially in investigating higher doses. However, our studies convinced us that normal human subjects cannot tolerate a higher dose on a continuing basis; and in fact, this was confirmed during the present study: when the codes were broken, it was found that there had been a number of complaints of side effects such as grogginess on 50 mg per day of chlorpromazine. Thus, although 50 mg per day is a low dose in clinical terms, it is apparently the maximum dose tolerable for continued use by normal subjects. The dosage range could have been extended only in the direction of lower doses which would have been of less interest. We found the same problems with reserpine, chloral hydrate, and amitriptyline.

The statistical analysis also could have been done in many different ways. We have restricted ourselves chiefly to visual representation of time-curves and to simple *t*-tests and correlation coefficients in areas of interest. An attempt was made to apply other statistical measures such as multivariate analysis, and various time series analyses, but it did not appear that these would be useful in the overall presentation of these data.

Another issue is just how seriously to take any result which reaches statistical significance in a large multivariable study such as this. This problem is not so serious in the simple drug versus placebo comparisons as in the large correlation matrices relating variables to one another. We have tended on the whole to be conservative, especially in the correlations, and to mention results only when a group of related comparisons reached significance at $p < 0.05$ or when specific single comparisons reached significance at higher levels. In the correlation matrices we have tried to present enough data so that the reader can to some extent make up his own mind. Due to the large number of correlation coefficients obtained, it is not acceptable merely to take a single probability at face value. On the other hand, a procedure of reducing levels of significance by taking into account the number of tests performed is not suitable either; this would lead to considerable type 2 errors, since the very large number of correlation coefficients obtained was an artifact: it was easier to direct the computer to print out a complete correlation matrix than only the specific correlations in which we might have been interested.

RESULTS: THE EFFECTS OF PLACEBO ON SLEEP

The placebo ("I shall please") is an important agent in medicine and somewhat deceptively named. There have now been a large number of studies of placebo effect on various physiological and behavioral measures which cannot be reviewed in detail here; clearly, placebo administration sometimes has a variety of effects, negative as well as positive—for instance, there are reports involving side effects of placebo administration (Shader and DiMascio, 1970). Such findings are of course responsible for the widespread and very reasonable trend at present to compare a drug to a similar-appearing placebo whenever one wishes to determine the specific pharmacological effect of the drug, as opposed to its total effect (which would include placebo effect) on the patient.

There has been little investigation so far of the direct effects of placebo on sleep. In most sleep studies in which placebo is employed, it is used on all non-drug nights, or sometimes all non-drug nights except for the first one or two "adaptation" nights. With such a design it is impossible directly to compare placebo nights with similar non-placebo nights, since placebo effect would be confounded with adaptation effect.

One drug study in our laboratory employed a design in which sleep was studied approximately one night per week with no medication and certain subjects then received placebo on their sixth or seventh such night (Hartmann, 1967). There was a trend, not quite reaching significance levels, towards a decrease of D-time and an increased number of awakenings on the first placebo night. In other words, the first placebo night showed a recurrence of some of the characteristics of the first night in the laboratory.

In a recent study we specifically investigated the effects of no medication, placebo, and an over-the-counter sleeping medication, Sominex (Davis and Hartmann, 1973). In this study, after an adaptation night, each subject slept in the laboratory nine nights; three nights on each of the three conditions in a balanced design. Two studies were done, one on the usual group of young male volunteers, age 21–35, and the other on a group of women, age 45–60, who are the greatest consumers of over-the-counter sleeping medications. Here placebo and no medication can be directly compared. Interestingly, in the young males sleep was "worse" on placebo than on no medication in a number of ways; time awake was significantly greater on placebo than no medication, and sleep latency was longer. D-time tended to be lower and D-latency longer on placebo although these did not reach significance. However, in the women of 45–60, sleep appeared somewhat "better" on placebo than on no medication: the number of D-periods, amount of stage 3 and of slow-wave sleep were significantly higher on placebo. Waking time was somewhat less, sleep time higher, D-time higher, and D-latency lower (N.S.).

These studies suggest that there are interesting individual differences in placebo effect, perhaps most easily explainable in terms of expectations of the medication. Thus, in our groups the older women may have had a positive expectation that any medication tested in a sleep laboratory might help them sleep, even though they were not specifically told this. On the other hand, young male subjects often tend to dislike the idea of taking sleeping medication, so that placebo effect for them can be quite different.

In any case, the present study affords the first opportunity to look at long-term placebo effects, i.e., the effects of the initial administration of placebo, long-term continuing placebo administration, and discontinuation of placebo. We have an opportunity to compare this long placebo period with the drug-free baseline period (no medication) in the same subjects; this will also give some indication of whether nights 3–6 are an adequate representation of a subject's eventual sleep pattern.

The overall comparison between means for the entire placebo period and the baseline period (nights 3–6 or 4–6) are presented in Table 2. It can be seen that there is a significant difference in one variable, D-time, and the related variable, D-time as a percent of sleep. D-time is significantly higher overall during the two months on and off placebo period than during baseline.

Fig. 2 presents the mean and standard error of the mean for sleep time plotted over the entire two-month on-and-off placebo experimental period in the 12 subjects who completed the placebo period. This curve is compared to baseline mean ± S.E.M. for the same subjects. Figs. 3 and 4 present similar graphs for SWS and for D-time. Slow-wave sleep time (Fig. 3) shows no obvious effect on placebo administration or discontinuation; placebo values are always close to baseline. However, D-time, and to a lesser extent, total sleep show

Table 2. Baseline versus placebo

	Baseline mean $N = 14$	Placebo mean $N = 12$	Mean diff. $N = 12$
Waking time (30 sec pages)	54.8	40.5	18.6
Number of awakenings	3.6	2.7	0.9
Sleep latency (30 sec pages)	24.2	22.0	5.8
Total sleep time (30 sec pages)	818	837	−19.3
Stage 1 (30 sec pages)	35.9	34.5	3.7
Stage 2 (30 sec pages)	433	434	− 0.4
Stage 3 (30 sec pages)	68.6	64.2	3.7
Stage 4 (30 sec pages)	81.8	86.1	3.0
Slow-wave sleep (30 sec pages)	150	150	6.6
D-time (30 sec pages)	199	219	−29.0***
D per cent	24.4	25.8	− 2.8**
D latency (30 sec pages)	184	170	19.0
Number of D-periods	4.1	4.0	0.0
Stage shifts	54.4	56.3	− 0.7
Cycle length (30 sec pages)	208	206	0.7
Body movements	45.3	49.2	− 2.7
Disturbance index	100.0	89.7	15.8

* $P < 0.05$; ** $P < 0.01$; *** $P < 0.005$. Mean diff.-baseline minus placebo, for 12 subjects.

some interesting changes: there is no dramatic effect when placebo is first given, but several days after discontinuation of placebo there is a distinct increase in D-time and a small but significant increase in total sleep as well. Overall D-time is higher on placebo than during baseline, and at a number of time points significantly higher.

DISCUSSION

There are two major questions to be discussed. First of all, the question of what light these results shed on *adaptation* to the sleep laboratory. There is a type of sleep characteristic of the first night in the laboratory usually involving somewhat less sleep and more awakenings than on later nights and a definitely low D-time (Agnew et al., 1967; Hartmann, 1967). These, and especially the characteristically reduced D-time, have become known as the

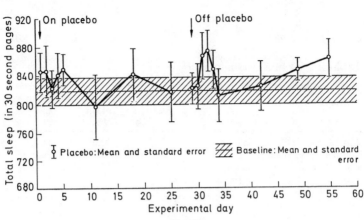

Fig. 2

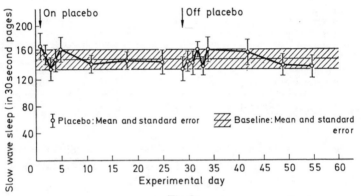

Fig. 3

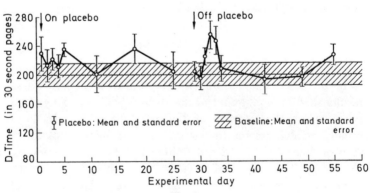

Fig. 4

"first night effect." Unfortunately, though fairly obviously, one cannot expect this "first night effect" always to be restricted to the first night, and we have noted that in some subjects, especially anxious ones, the second, third, and fourth nights may still show some of these characteristics. Dement (1964) has reported that in a few subjects D-time may still be increasing after 8–10 consecutive nights in the laboratory.

What we have shown here, in terms of adaptation effect, is that this process may still be going on, at least with regard to the variable D-time, for a period of months. Thus the mean total D-time and mean D-time percent for the entire placebo period is significantly higher than in the baseline period (nights 3–6). Ten of the 12 subjects had higher D-time on placebo than on "baseline." This must be kept in mind for future drug studies, and it emphasizes the importance of using balanced or crossover designs whenever possible rather than comparing results in a series of drug nights with a series of earlier placebo nights.

The other question is the effect of placebo itself—short-term or long-term administration of a placebo, or its discontinuation—on sleep variables. To examine this question individual points on the placebo time-curve can be compared to mean baseline, to mean placebo values, or to the late off-placebo points, when no medication has been taken for 3–5 weeks. Looking at the curves in Figs. 3 and 4 shows that D-time appears more responsive or changeable than slow-wave sleep. As mentioned, the greatest change is the increased D-time several days after placebo discontinuation. The results do not suggest any obvious explanation, but our impression from these subjects is that the nights after discontinuation of medication, especially several nights thereafter, were sometimes associated with feeling better, with feeling they were "over the hump," and nearing the end of one more drug study period. Thus, here the increased D-time and somewhat increased sleep could be associated with feeling better or more relaxed.

The placebo curves will be noted and discussed again in

terms of the individual drug results to be presented in later papers. Having obtained this long-term placebo data will obviously be useful, for instance, in preventing us from being overly impressed by a "rebound increase" in D-time after drug discontinuation, especially if it coincides fairly closely with the time-curve of increase on placebo.

This work was supported in part by National Institute of Mental Health Grant # MH 14520.

Bibliography

Agnew, H. W., Webb, W. B., Williams, R. L.: The first night effect: An EEG study. Electroenceph. clin. Neurophysiol. **23,** 168–171 (1967)

Brodman, K., Erdmann, A. J., Lorge, J., Wolff, H. C., Broadbent, T. H.: The Cornell Medical Index: An adjunct to medical interviewing. J. Amer. med. Ass. **140,** 530 (1949)

Dement, W. C.: Experimental dream studies. In: Development and research. J. H. Masserman, ed. Science and psychoanalysis, vol. 7, pp. 129–161. New York: Grune & Stratton 1964

Hartmann, E.: Dreaming sleep (the D-state) and the menstrual cycle. J. nerv. ment. Dis. **143,** 406–416 (1966)

Hartmann, E.: Adaptation to the sleep laboratory and placebo effect. (Report to the Association for the Psychophysiological Study of Sleep, Santa Monica, California, April 1967.) Abstract: Psychophysiology **4,** 389 (1967)

Hartmann, E.: Amitriptyline and imipramine. Effects on human sleep. (Report to the Association for the Psychophysiological Study of Sleep, Denver, Colorado, March 1968.) Abstract: Psychophysiology **5,** 207 (1968a)

Hartmann, E.: The effect of four drugs on sleep in man. Psychopharmacologia (Berl.) **12,** 346–353 (1968b)

Hartmann, E.: The biochemistry and pharmacology of the D-state (dreaming sleep) In: Drugs and dreams—Proceedings of the Carl Neuberg Society for International Scientific Relations, Philadelphia: March 29–30, 1967). Exp. Med. Surg. **27,** 105–120 (1969)

Hartmann, E., Cravens, J.: The effects of long term administration of psychotropic drugs on human sleep. V. The effects of chloral hydrate. Psychopharmacologia (Berl.) **33**, 219–232 (1973)

Hartmann, E., Cravens, J., List, S.: L-Tryptophan as a natural hypnotic: A dose-response study in man. Report to the Association for the Psychophysiological Study of Sleep, San Diego, May 1973

Hartmann, E., Davis, D.: A comparison of the effects of an OTC sleeping medication, placebo, and no medication on human sleep. Report to the Association for the Psychophysiological Study of Sleep, San Diego, May 1973

Kales, A., Allen, C., Scharf, M. B., Kales, J. D.: Hypnotic drugs and their effectiveness: All-night EEG studies of insomniac subjects. Arch. gen. Psychiat. **23**, 226–232 (1970)

Kales, A., Kales, J. D., Scharf, M. B., Tan, T.-L.: Hypnotics and altered sleep-dream patterns. 2. All-night EEG studies of chloral hydrate, flurazepam, and methaqualone. Arch. gen. Psychiat. **23**, 219–225 (1970)

Kales, A., Malmstram, E. J., Kee, H. K., Kales, J. D., Tan, T.-L.: Effects of hypnotics on sleep patterns, dreaming, and mood state—Laboratory and home studies. Biol. Psychiat. **1**, 235–241 (1969)

Kales, A., Preston, T. A., Tan, T.-L., Allen, C.: Hypnotics and altered sleep-dream patterns. 1. All-night EEG studies of flutethimide, methyprylon, and pentobarbital. Arch. gen. Psychiat. **23**, 211–218 (1970)

Lana, R. E., Lubin, A.: The effect of correlation on the repeated measures design. Educ. Psychol. Measmt. **23**, 729–739 (1963)

McNair, D. M., Lorr, M., Droppleman, L. F.: Profile of Mood States (Manual), San Diego, Educ. & Indus. Testing Serv. (1971)

Rechtschaffen, A., Kales, A., eds. with Berger, R. J., Dement, W. C., Jacobson, A., Johnson, L. C., Jouvet, M., Monroe, L. J., Oswald, I., Roffward, H. P., Roth, B., Walter, R. D.: A Manual for Standardized Terminology, Techniques and Scoring System for Sleep Stages of Human Subjects. Wash. D.C.: Publ. Health Serv. U.S. Govt. Print. Off. (1968), Publication No. 204

Rotter, J. B., Willerman, B.: The incomplete sentence test as a method of studying personality. J. cons. Psychol. **11**, 43 (1947)

Shader, R. I., DiMascio, A. (eds.): Psychotropic drug side effects: Clinical and theoretical perspectives. Baltimore: Williams & Wilkins 1970

The Effects of Long-Term Administration of Psychotropic Drugs on Human Sleep: The Effects of Amitriptyline

Ernest Hartmann and James Cravens

Sleep and Dream Laboratory, Boston State Hospital, Department of Psychiatry, Tufts University School of Medicine

Abstract. This paper reports on the effects of the daily administration of amitriptyline (50 mg) to normal young males. Effects on laboratory recorded sleep, home sleep, and mood were studied. Total sleep time was significantly increased throughout administration, while slow-wave sleep was increased and sleep latency decreased early during administration. D-time and D-time percent were decreased throughout administration, most prominently for the first days; there was a "rebound" increase after discontinuation of medication.

In these subjects, amitriptyline did not alter "depression" as measured by mood scales, but did produce a number of different complaints in the morning.

Amitriptyline is now perhaps the most widely used clinical antidepressant agent. It is one of the more recently developed tricyclic antidepressants, and has effects on depression similar or slightly superior to those of imipramine and the monoamine oxidase inhibitors, with relatively few side effects (Burt et al., 1962; Hordern et al., 1963; Klerman and Cole, 1965).

Although the mechanism by which antidepressant effects are produced is not absolutely established, the most widely held view relates the antidepressant action to the effects on central catecholamines. The tricyclic antidepressants, including amitriptyline, apparently increase the metabolism of catecholamines, especially norepinephrine, through the O-methylation pathways (Schildkraut et al., 1971, 1972). Since O-methylation is the enzymatic reaction thought to occur with extracellular, probably synaptically released, transmitters, this suggests that more norepinephrine or dopamine is available at the synapses after tricyclic antidepressants. The mechanism by which this increased availability at the synapses is produced may be the prevention of reuptake of the catecholamines, especially by presynaptic neurons (Glowinski and Axelrod, 1964). However, this mechanism is not certain, and some studies have shown that amitriptyline does not have this specific action in blocking reuptake, so that amitriptyline may produce a similar increase in synaptically available catecholamines by some other mechanism (Schildkraut et al., 1969; Stille, 1968). Amitriptyline does prevent reuptake and increase the turnover of central serotonin (Carlsson et al., 1969 a, 1969 b; Himwich and Alpers, 1970); this mechanism may well be involved in the antidepressants effect rather than or in addition to the effect on the catecholamines.

Overall, the tricyclic antidepressants, acting by different mechanisms, produce a somewhat similar end result as the MAO inhibitors, i.e., an increase in availability of biogenic amines at central synapses. These drugs cannot be used to differentiate clearly between the various biogenic amines—dopamine, norepinephrine, and serotonin—since somewhat similar effects are produced on each.

Amitriptyline is of special interest to us for several reasons aside from its wide clinical use. Since its effects on depression and its effects on the biogenic amines seem in many ways exactly opposite to those of reserpine, it is of interest to examine whether the effects on sleep or the effects on certain parameters of sleep may also be opposite. In fact, results of short-term studies do indicate that the antidepressant drugs produce a marked decrease in the amount of desynchronized sleep (D-time) accompanied by great increase in D-latency (Hartmann, 1968 a; Wyatt et al., 1969; Zung, 1969 a; Akindele et al., 1970), an effect opposite to the results with reserpine

(Hartmann, 1966; Hoffman and Domino, 1969; Coulter et al., 1971).

There is no question in the literature about the initial effects of amitriptyline in decreasing D-time, but the present long-term investigation should allow us to resolve a controversy in the literature as to long-term effects of amitriptyline and as to whether or not there is a rebound increase in D-time after discontinuation of medication.

In addition to its principal antidepressant effects already discussed, amitriptyline appears definitely to have soporific or sleep-inducing effects on its own (Dobkin et al., 1963; Allen and Bonica, 1965; Urbach, 1967) greater than any found with the MAO inhibitors or imipramine. The biochemical mechanisms for this effect are not established. These studies will allow us to examine and determine the time-course of this sleep-inducing effect of amitriptyline.

There have been few previous studies on amitriptyline itself. We have shown in a short-term human study that D-time is clearly decreased and D-latency greatly increased on initial administration of amitriptyline. There was a trend towards increase in total sleep, but no change in sleep latency (Hartmann, 1968 a, 1968 b).

There have been a number of studies of the effects of other antidepressants on recorded sleep. Generally these have been either single-dose studies or very short-term studies in normal subjects, although there have been a few longer studies in depressed patients which are somewhat difficult to evaluate: Desipramine, in normal subjects, produced no change in amount of total sleep; there was some decrease in slow-wave sleep and decrease in stage shifts; D-time was decreased by about 50% (Zung, 1969 a); MAO inhibitors, studied chiefly in depressed patients or occasionally in a subject taking an overdose, tend to produce a gradual decrease in D-time without dramatic effects on total sleep or slow-wave sleep (Wyatt et al., 1969; Cramer and Kuhlo, 1967; Ryba et al., 1966). It has recently been shown that long-term administration of large doses of MAO inhibitors in depressed patients can reduce D-time to zero for a period of months (Wyatt et al., 1971 b).

A recent study has shown differential sleep effects with different tricyclic antidepressants (Dunleavy et al., 1972). It is interesting that whereas most antidepressants produced the decrease in D-time mentioned, two of them—iprindole and trimipramine—were not associated with a decrease in D-time. These are preliminary studies, however, and also it is not certain that these two drugs are effective antidepressants.

Studies of the effects of antidepressants on sleep in hospitalized depressed patients (Zung, 1969 b; Akindele et al., 1970; Wyatt et al., 1971) have shown decreased stage shifts over a long period, during a time of generally "improved" sleep. Our laboratory has been involved in such studies as well; we have often found increased sleep as well as decreased D-time; however, these studies are difficult to evaluate in terms of a primary effect of amitriptyline, since the period of amitriptyline administration often coincides with a period of clinical improvement, and often with a period of recovery from previous sleep deprivation.

Animal studies of the MAO inhibitors and the tricyclic antidepressants have also found the decrease in D-time; other effects on sleep are less clear (Jouvet et al., 1965; Khazan and Sawyer, 1964; Khazan and Sulman, 1966; Wallach et al., 1969). Sometimes a "rebound" increase in D-time has been found after the initial decrease produced by these drugs, but there has been some difference of opinion on this point. Studies in the cat (Jouvet et al., 1965; Wallach et al., 1969) and our human studies (Hartmann, 1968 b) appeared first to show no rebound increase or a very delayed rebound. The present long-term study should be able to settle these differences.

It is of interest that the reported effects on sleep are immediate whereas the effects on depression of all of these antidepressants sometimes take a week to two weeks to develop; it will be of interest in this long-term study to examine differential effects on sleep after a one- to two-week period, to

see whether any changes occur at the time when clinical
effects appear.

Long-term studies of amitriptyline may be of additional
interest because it has at times been suggested by physicians
treating insomnia, including our own group, that some insomniacs may have the "sleep characteristics" of depression
even when they are not overtly depressed and that antidepressants may constitute a specific treatment for this insomnia.
Present studies would at least give a baseline, an expectation
of what effects are produced in normal subjects on long-term
administration, against which long-term effects on insomniacs
may then be compared.

The present design allows us to examine not only the effects
on laboratory sleep, but the effects on subjective aspects of
sleep, on mood, and on daily activities. This may shed some
light on the question of whether amitriptyline has antidepressant properties only in certain severely depressed patients,
or whether the chemical changes it produces will push even
normal individuals towards filling out less of the "depressive"
adjectives on subjective mood forms.

METHODS

The methodology for this long-
term study has been discussed in great detail in the first paper
of this series (Hartmann and Cravens, 1973). Briefly, 14 subjects were studied for a total of 1,125 nights of recorded
laboratory sleep. Subjects were normal males age 21–35. The
design for each subject included six 60-day study periods, one
for each of the following drug conditions in a balanced
design: placebo; reserpine 0.50 mg daily; amitriptyline 50 mg
daily; chlorpromazine 50 mg daily; chloral hydrate 500 mg
daily; and chlordiazepoxide 50 mg daily. Subjects, experimenters who ran the studies at night, and assistants who
scored the records were all blind to drug condition.

During each 60-day period, the subject took a single pink
capsule (drug or placebo) 20 min before bedtime every night
for 28 nights, and then no medication for approximately 32

nights. Subjects slept in the laboratory the first five nights on medication, then once a week for the remainder of the medication period, then the first six nights after discontinuation of medication, then once a week for the remainder of the discontinuation period. The laboratory nights in a single study period would be approximately 1, 2, 3, 4, 5, 12, 18, 25, 29, 30, 31, 32, 33, 34, 42, 49, 55. In addition to these 17 nights of uninterrupted sleep, each period includes one laboratory night during which the subject is awakened to study possible drug effect on dream content.

Subjects filled out a sleep log every morning throughout the study whether they slept at home or in the laboratory. They filled in time to bed, time up, estimate of time slept, any dreams, any unusual events or side effects, and then were asked to rate on a simple 5-point scale both the quality of their sleep for the night and how they felt that morning. Subjects filled out a adjective checklist—the Psychiatric Outpatient Mood Scale (POMS)—once per week throughout the study, and were instructed to answer the questions for the entire past week, i.e., how they had tended to feel that week, not how they were feeling at the time they filled out the form.

A total of ten subjects completed the two-month study period on amitriptyline, and of these all ten completed both amitriptyline and placebo periods. The statistical comparisons relating amitriptyline and placebo below refer to within-subject comparisons on these ten subjects who completed both drug conditions. Thus, for instance, a comparison of amitriptyline versus placebo for the first five days on medication involves obtaining the mean value for each variable on amitriptyline, and then the mean values on placebo for a given subject; measures of difference are then handled across subjects by t-tests for correlated samples.

RESULTS

Effects of Amitriptyline on Laboratory Sleep. Table 1 presents overall results on the effects of amitriptyline for the time periods of interest to us. In

Table 1. Amitriptyline: Effects on laboratory sleep

	On medication					Off medication				
	First night	First 3 nights	First 5 nights	Remaining nights	All nights	First night	First 3 nights	Second 3 nights	Remaining nights	Last night
Time awake (30-sec pages)	29.2 (−16.6)	30.4 (−18.6)	34.7 (−15.0)	40.7 (+2.2)	36.9 (−7.9)	50.8 (+0.4)	58.3 (+19.7)*	58.4 (+19.8)*	45.9 (−4.2)	38.3 (−8.3)
Number of awakenings	3.3 (+0.3)	3.6 (+0.4)	4.0 (+1.0)	3.5 (+1.1)	3.8 (+1.0)	4.5 (+1.6)	4.7 (+1.3)	3.7 (+0.6)	2.4 (−0.6)	1.3 (−1.3)
Sleep latency (30-sec pages)	20.4 (−3.5)	18.7 (−4.8)	19.1 (−2.8)	26.3 (+4.1)	21.8 (+0.2)	24.9 (+7.2)	27.1 (+7.3)*	23.3 (+2.0)	21.4 (−10.8)	16.7 (−14.1)
Total sleep time (30-sec pages)	874 (+28.5)	883 (+43.7)*	875 (+32.9)*	846 (+29.1)	864 (+27.0)	858 (+34.8)	855 (+17.3)	832 (−11.2)	836 (−3.9)	850 (−9.9)
Stage 1 (30-sec pages)	20.3 (−17.0)*	29.8 (−5.9)	33.8 (−3.4)	41.1 (+7.0)	36.6 (+0.4)	46.7 (+19.6)*	37.5 (+5.6)	38.6 (+8.6)*	30.8 (+0.6)	33.9 (+6.4)
Stage 2 (30-sec pages)	550 (+138.2)***	545 (+118.4)***	525 (+97.5)***	486 (+61.0)**	511 (+83.2)***	391 (−62.2)*	413 (−42.8)*	380 (−28.9)*	456 (+10.4)	475 (+39.2)
Stage 3 (30-sec pages)	121.0 (+30.1)	101.5 (+26.7)*	96.9 (+23.5)**	88.1 (+17.2)*	93.6 (+20.4)***	73.9 (−3.1)***	64.7 (−1.4)	67.2 (+3.6)	63.8 (−1.0)	65.1 (−2.1)
Stage 4 (30-sec pages)	91.9 (+16.6)	81.6 (−0.5)	81.7 (−2.4)	78.5 (+1.8)	80.5 (−1.0)	57.1 (−24.9)*	55.5 (−20.7)*	54.2 (−41.9)***	76.2 (−21.3)*	71.4 (−25.5)
Slow-wave sleep (30-sec pages)	213 (+46.7)	183 (+26.2)	179 (+21.1)	167 (+18.9)	174 (+19.4)	131 (−12.2)	120 (−22.1)*	121 (−38.3)***	140 (−22.3)*	136 (−27.6)

D-Time (30-sec pages)	91 (−139.4)***	124 (−95.1)***	137 (−82.4)***	153 (−57.7)*	143 (−76.0)***	289 (+89.6)***	284 (+76.6)***	291 (+47.4)*	209 (+15.2)	204 (−8.1)
D-Latency (30-sec pages)	294 (+125.0)	241 (+65.3)*	250 (+77.4)*	255 (+75.1)*	252 (+78.1)**	146 (−23.2)*	142 (−25.2)*	114 (−25.9)*	160 (−39.2)	186 (−33.8)
Number of D-periods	2.5 (−1.5)***	2.8 (−1.2)***	2.9 (−1.1)***	3.0 (−1.0)*	3.0 (−1.1)***	4.0 (+0.1)	4.2 (+0.3)	4.6 (+0.4)***	3.9 (+0.1)	3.9 (+0.3)
Number of stage shifts	61.2 (+6.8)	58.9 (+3.8)	60.4 (+5.0)	56.5 (+2.0)	59.0 (+3.6)	58.5 (+7.2)	57.3 (+3.7)	55.6 (+0.8)	52.6 (−1.4)	49.2 (−3.6)
Cycle length (30-sec pages)	260 (+46.3)	310 (+102.6)***	297 (+89.6)***	232 (+33.4)	272 (+68.8)***	228 (+13.2)	218 (+0.2)	197 (−12.5)	218 (+5.2)	212 (−15.3)
Number of body movements	48.5 (+1.4)	46.6 (−2.2)	45.9 (−2.6)	52.1 (+6.3)	48.2 (+0.7)	46.4 (−1.0)	48.9 (+1.3)	52.2 (+6.8)**	46.8 (−5.3)	53.8 (−3.8)
Disturbance index	77.7 (−15.2)	77.1 (−20.7)	80.6 (−17.6)	92.8 (+8.3)	85.2 (−7.2)	97.2 (−0.6)	107.2 (+21.0)**	110.6 (+26.6)**	92.7 (−9.4)	92.1 (−4.5)

* $P < 0.05$. ** $P < 0.01$. *** $P < 0.001$.

Figures in parentheses represent drug value minus placebo value.

Time awake. All waking from start to end of EEG recording; *Number of awakenings*: Number of periods of waking separated from other periods of waking by at least 5 min of sleep; *Sleep latency*: Time spent from start of recording until first Stage 1 which reaches Stage 2; *Total sleep time*: Sum of Stages 1–4 and REM; Stages 1–3, and 4; *D-time*: Time spent in Stage REM; *D-latency*: Total time *asleep* before the first occurrence of Stage REM; *Number of D-periods*: Number of occurrences of Stage REM separated by more than 15 min; *Number of Stage shifts*: Total number of Stage changes; *Cycle length*: Average time between ends of D-periods; *Number of body movements*: Number of body movements more than 5 sec in length; *Disturbance index*: Sum of number of body movements and time awake.

terms of overall sleep measures, amitriptyline produced an increase of about 15 min in total sleep (Fig. 1) throughout the period of administration, reaching significance for the first five nights on medication. It is important to remember that the total sleep time of these subjects was to a large extent shaped by their regular schedule—they had to go to work and had planned evening activities—so that even a small change in total sleep time must be considered unusual. There was a trend to decreased waking time, early in administration (not significant) with a clearly significant increase in waking time the first week off medication (Fig. 2). No change in number of awakenings, number of body movements or stage shifts was found.

Slow-wave sleep showed a tendency to increase during the medication period though the increase was mainly in stage 3 rather than in stage 4, followed by a clear and significant decrease in slow-wave sleep and in stage 4 during the first week off medication (Fig. 3).

D-time was strikingly decreased on initial administration of

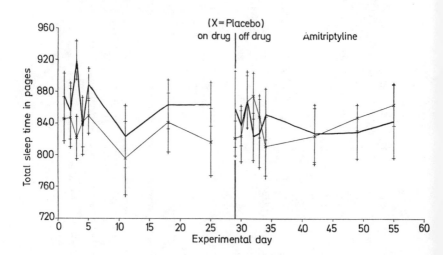

Fig. 1. Effect of amitriptyline on total sleep time

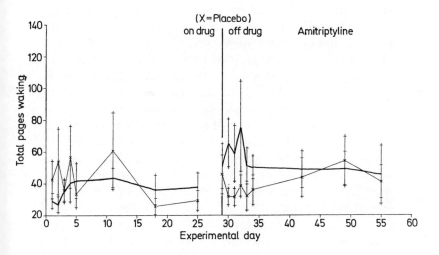

Fig. 2. Effect of amitriptyline on waking time

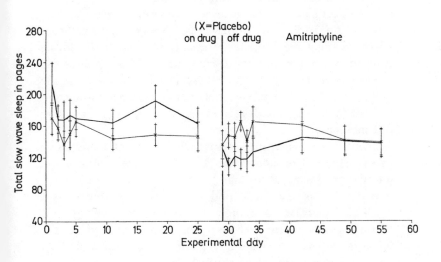

Fig. 3. Effect of amitriptyline on slow wave sleep

amitriptyline, rose somewhat during the next four days, but remained significantly below placebo values throughout the period of drug administration (a decrease of about 30% from placebo values) (Fig. 4). There was a clear increase in D-time over placebo values during the first six days after discontinuation of medication. The values returned to normal somewhere between the 6th and 14th day after discontinuation. D-time as a percent of sleep (Fig. 5), and the number of D-periods varied in the same way as D-time, with a great decrease at first, a lesser decrease continuing throughout administration and then a slight increase just after discontinuation. D-latency mirrored D-time with a significant increase on medication (highest when D-time was lowest) and then a decrease after discontinuation (Fig. 6). Sleep-dream cycle length was very significantly increased over all nights on medication and particularly on the first five nights when the increase averaged about 45 min.

Effects on Home Sleep Variables. Overall results are presented in Table 2. Amitriptyline produced an increase in the subjects' estimate of time asleep, reaching statistical significance on the first and third weeks. There was no significant effect on subjective estimates of quality of sleep either during drug administration or after discontinuation. Amitriptyline did produce significantly lower ratings (feeling worse) on the question of how the subject felt in the morning throughout the first three weeks of drug administration, but not after drug discontinuation.

There were significant increases in reports of feeling sick (weeks 3 and 4 on and weeks 1 and 2 off medication) and unusual psychological feelings (week 4 on medication). More importantly, on weeks 2, 3, and 4 on medication there was a significant increase in number of complaints (feeling sick, unusual psychological feelings) which were blamed on the medication. This is a much larger number of complaints than with the other medications studied.

There was a significant increase in the "fatigue" factor on the POMS scale. This was present throughout the period of administration, and continued for a week after discontinuation.

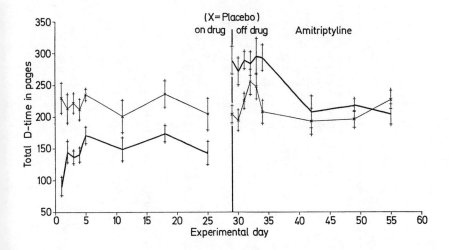

Fig. 4. Effect of amitriptyline on D-time

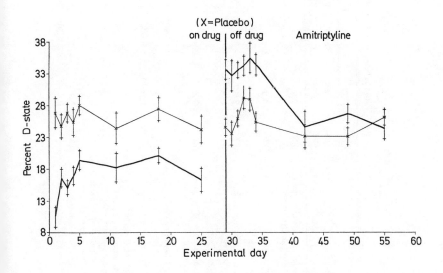

Fig. 5. Effect of amitriptyline on D-time as a percent of total sleep

Table 2. Amitriptyline: Effects on home log variables

	On medication					Off medication				
	First week	Second week	Third week	Fourth week	All weeks	First week	Second week	Third week	Fourth week	All weeks
Estimated total sleep time (in hours and tenths)	8.2 (+ 0.7)**	7.8 (+ 0.1)	7.9 (+ 0.5)*	6.6 (+ 0.5)	7.9 (+ 0.4)	7.0 (− 0.6)	7.5 (− 0.3)	6.6 (− 0.2)	6.6 (+ 0.7)	7.3 (− 0.3)
Quality of sleep (1 = worst to 5 = best)	3.0 (+ 0.1)	3.0 (+ 0.0)	2.9 (− 0.1)	2.8 (+ 0.4)	3.0 (+ 0.0)	2.9 (− 0.0)	2.9 (− 0.1)	2.7 (+ 0.2)*	2.7 (+ 0.3)	3.0 (+ 0.0)
How feel in the morning (1 = worst to 5 = best)	2.7 (− 0.2)*	2.6 (− 0.3)***	2.7 (− 0.3)*	2.4 (− 0.0)	2.7 (− 0.3)***	2.9 (− 0.0)	2.8 (− 0.0)	2.5 (+ 0.0)	2.6 (+ 0.4)	2.9 (+ 0.0)
Feel sick in any way (mean number of positive responses)	0.4 (+ 0.2)	0.2 (− 0.0)	0.3 (+ 0.2)*	0.4 (+ 0.4)*	0.3 (+ 0.2)*	0.1 (+ 0.1)*	0.1 (+ 0.1)*	0.1 (+ 0.0)	0.1 (+ 0.0)	0.1 (+ 0.1)
Unusual psychological feelings (mean number of positive responses)	0.1 (+ 0.0)	0.2 (+ 0.1)	0.2 (+ 0.2)	0.3 (+ 0.3)*	0.2 (+ 0.1)	0.2 (+ 0.2)	0.1 (− 0.0)	0.0 (− 0.1)	0.0 (− 0.1)	0.1 (− 0.0)
Fault of medication (mean number of positive responses—this refers to the two immediately preceding items and was only answered if there was a positive response to either)	0.3 (+ 0.1)	0.3 (+ 0.3)*	0.3 (+ 0.3)*	0.4 (+ 0.4)*	0.5 (+ 0.3)*	0.2 (+ 0.2)	0.0 (− 0.0)	0.0 (+ 0.0)	0.0 (+ 0.0)	0.2 (+ 0.2)

Psychiatric outpatient
mood scale:

Tension-anxiety	-3.2 (-1.2)	-2.5 (+0.6)	-1.2 (+0.5)	-0.8 (+0.7)	-2.2 (+0.1)	-1.9 (-0.4)	-2.4 (-0.9)	-1.4 (+0.9)	-2.2 (+0.5)	-1.9 (-0.6)
Anger-hostility	-10.5 (-0.5)	-9.2 (+1.4)	-7.5 (+1.5)	-5.1 (+2.6)	-8.8 (+1.2)	-6.9 (+0.4)	-8.8 (-1.8)	-6.5 (-0.3)	-6.2 (-0.6)	-7.5 (-0.9)
Fatigue	0.5 (-6.0)*	1.0 (+6.3)*	1.0 (+6.8)**	1.7 (+5.6)*	1.0 (+6.5)**	-1.6 (+3.1)**	-4.5 (-1.0)	-3.8 (+0.1)	-4.2 (+0.1)	-3.8 (+0.2)
Depression	-12.2 (-2.0)	-11.8 (-1.5)	-10.4 (-0.5)	-8.7 (-1.8)	-11.3 (-1.2)	-9.8 (-1.8)	-11.6 (-5.0)	-9.0 (-0.3)	-10.1 (-1.3)	-10.5 (-2.5)
Vigor	6.5 (-1.9)	5.4 (-2.9)	4.5 (-2.9)	3.7 (+1.2)	5.3 (-2.2)	6.4 (+2.1)	8.6 (+2.7)*	8.5 (+2.0)	4.2 (-3.2)	6.9 (+1.1)
Confusion	-0.3 (+0.0)	-0.4 (-0.2)	0.6 (-0.4)	1.0 (+0.1)	-0.0 (-0.3)	-0.0 (-1.3)	-0.7 (-1.6)	-0.6 (+0.8)	-1.8 (-0.3)	-0.6 (-1.8)

* $P < 0.05$.   ** $P < 0.01$.   *** $P < 0.001$.

Figures in parentheses represent drug value minus placebo value.

Home Log Variables. Except for the *POMS* (Psychiatric Outpatient Mood Scale), home log variables are from daily responses in diaries kept by each subject. The *POMS* consists of an adjective check list filled in weekly. Subjects were asked to consider their feeling for the entire week, not just that day.

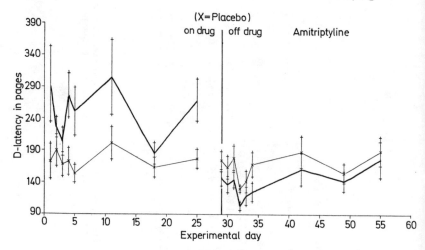

Fig. 6. Effect of amitriptyline on D-latency

The other POMS mood variables, including "depression," showed no significant change on medication.

Effects on Interrelationships between Laboratory Variables.
A night of sleep generally demonstrates certain consistency, or a kind of coherence between laboratory sleep variables. Some of the interrelationships between laboratory variables very reliably found on placebo were clearly altered on amitriptyline. Amitriptyline produced more changes than any other of the drugs studied on this sort of measure of coherence or interrelation. For instance, on placebo there is always a very high correlation between total sleep and total D-time $(r = + .68)$. On amitriptyline the correlation between total sleep and D-time was reduced to $+ 0.036$. On placebo there is a strong positive relationship $(r = + 0.41)$ between total D-time and total body movements; this is explainable on the basis of body movements typically occurring in D-time and especially at the beginnings and ends of the D-periods. The correlation is $+ 0.04$ on amitriptyline. Again, on placebo slow-wave sleep shows a negative correlation to stage 2 of $- 0.46$. This is a negative relation we have found on a number of studies. On amitriptyline this relationship is reduced to $- 0.17$. On the other hand, on placebo and in the overall study, slow-wave

sleep and total sleep show a close to zero correlation; on amitriptyline this correlation increases to + 0.42.

In other words, although the individual details are hard to explain, amitriptyline produces a considerable distortion of the normal interrelationships between laboratory variables, a distortion greater than that produced by other drugs and apparently not restricted to interrelationships involving D-time, in which amitriptyline produced a great change. Correlation coefficients between all laboratory and home variables were also examined. Some distortions were produced by amitriptyline in the usual relationships, but here amitriptyline did not so clearly differ from the other medication studied.

DISCUSSION

First of all, amitriptyline did not act as an "antidepressant" in this study: i.e., it did not decrease the POMS "depression" factor nor did it increase the "vigor" or "anger-hostility" factors on the POMS. No definite conclusions can be drawn, since these may not be very sensitive measures of depression in normal subjects; furthermore, the drowsiness and other side effects noted by the subjects on amitriptyline could have increased the scores on the depression factor. Thus one study (Oswald et al., 1972) showed that imipramine produced a "depressed mood" for a number of days in normal subjects. Possibly the lack of change seen here could be a resultant of a "depressive" effect related to the side effects, combined with some more positive effect of the drug.

Amitriptyline obviously produced profound changes in laboratory sleep patterns, as well as in the interrelationships between laboratory variables. First of all, sleep time was increased by about 15 min throughout drug administration; this is a considerable increase in normal subjects, who routinely slept 417 min out of 437 min in bed and frequently had morning commitments to keep. The most striking effect of amitriptyline was, of course, the profound depression of D-time with a clear increase after discontinuation. The effect was

in the opposite direction from that of reserpine, but the curves
do not show any very obvious day-to-day mirroring. In fact,
comparison of the two curves reveals amitriptyline had a
clearly longer-lasting effect—the decrease in D-time continued
throughout the period of drug administration. The two curves
for D-latency could be considered more nearly opposite in
that there was a great initial decrease in latency lasting 2 to
3 weeks on reserpine and an opposite effect, i.e., an increase
lasting 2 to 3 weeks on amitriptyline.

It may be of importance that a subject apparently adapts to
the effects of reserpine after one to two weeks but does not
show adaptation or tolerance to the opposite effects of amitriptyline even after four weeks. It is too early to try to link
these changes directly to chemical changes in biogenic amines
or other mechanisms produced by long-term administration of
these drugs.

The changes described in sleep parameters were generally
immediate and often lasted throughout the period of drug
administration as mentioned. There was no sleep variable
which changed dramatically at around one to two weeks, the
time when amitriptyline manifests its antidepressant effects
clinically; however, there were several variables that showed
at least some change. Slow-wave sleep (Fig. 3) was slightly
high early during drug administration but rose to a level
significantly above placebo levels (96 min versus 74 min)
only on the third week (day 18). Also, sleep latency was
slightly decreased for the first two weeks and then crossed the
placebo curve and was slightly increased for the remainder
of the period on amitriptyline, with a significant increase after
discontinuation (Fig. 7). Total waking showed a similar time-
course. There is no compelling reason at present to associate
these changes with antidepressant effect, but it is of interest
that, if anything, it was variables associated with sleep as a
whole or with SWS rather than D-time that showed these
third-week changes. Also, the overall sleep situation during
the third week on amitriptyline was unusual in that SWS was
high while sleep latency and waking time were also high,
while over the entire study and on placebo, SWS showed a

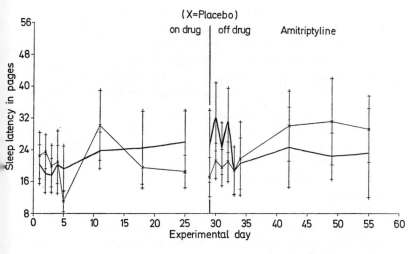

Fig. 7. Effects of amitriptyline on sleep latency

significantly negative relationship ($r = -0.2$ to -0.5) with these variables.

Trying to compare amitriptyline with other antidepressants is not simple since no other antidepressant has been studied in normal subjects in a similarly designed study. Comparisons with studies by others (Dunleavy et al., 1972; Zung, 1969 a; Wyatt et al., 1971) as well as our previous studies (Hartmann, 1968 a, 1968 b) suggest that the effects of amitriptyline are somewhat similar to those of imipramine and the MAO inhibitors, except that amitriptyline produces a slight increase in sleep time and a decrease in sleep latency. In other words, as previously suggested, amitriptyline appears to have more hypnotic effects, evident especially during the first days of administration. The fact that tolerance develops quickly to the sleep-inducing effect but not to the D-reducing effect possibly indicates that two quite separate brain mechanisms are involved.

In terms of clinical relationships, the sleep patterns of these normal subjects on long-term amitriptyline are reminiscent of two other groups we have studied: manic patients (Hartmann, 1968 c) and "short sleepers" (Hartmann et al., 1971), the latter being a group of normal subjects who always slept less than 6 hours per night and in terms of personality were found to be non-worriers, deniers, and in fact, slightly hypomanic. These subjects on amitriptyline did not, of course, have reduced total sleep time so that there is no relationship in this sense. However, the low D-time and D-time percent, combined with the normal or slightly high slow-wave sleep time is characteristic in our experience of both of these groups. Thus, although there was no detectable antidepressant effect attributable to the drug, nonetheless the subjects' sleep showed certain similarities to that of persons who tend to be manic or hypomanic.

Vogel demonstrated that some depressed patients are improved by one to two weeks of nightly D-deprivation (Vogel et al., 1968). He suggests that the antidepressants may work similarly by producing increased "D-pressure" and that the build-up of pressure over 1 to 2 weeks can explain the delayed action of these drugs. This study does not lend support to the hypothesis: increased D-pressure as seen during prolonged mechanical D-deprivation is demonstrated by decreased D-latency, increased number of D-periods and decreased cycle length, and a "rebound" increase in D-time on recovery nights. Only the last of these, the "rebound" increase, was found here, and even that was not especially impressive in amount; apparently, greater relative rebound increases are found after amphetamines and barbiturates (Oswald, 1971) and after alcohol (Gross and Goodenough, 1968; Greenberg and Pearlman, 1967), although the conditions of administration were not entirely comparable. Of course, the present subjects were not depressed and were taking less than the usual clinical dosage of amitriptyline, so that these results are not necessarily relevant to Vogel's hypothesis.

Clinically, the first week after discontinuation of amitriptyline should be considered carefully. During this first week there is a highly significant increase in waking time, tendency to increased body movements, increase in sleep latency, decrease in slow-wave sleep, increase in D-time, number of D-periods, and decrease in D-latency, and it is a time when relationships between laboratory variables are severely distorted. All these effects occurred in carefully screened young normal males on a dosage of only 0.50 mg per day, so that one might well expect larger effects in patients when a larger dose is suddenly withdrawn. One might expect considerable nocturnal discomfort, nightmares, and the possibility of exacerbation of conditions such as cardiac arrythmias, angina pectoris, peptic ulcer, and other conditions shown to be associated with D-periods at night (Nowlin et al., 1965; Armstrong et al., 1965; Rosenblatt et al., 1973). Clinically this finding would support the recommendation that amitriptyline be discontinued in small steps.

Concerning the possible use of amitriptyline in treating insomnia, this study cannot, of course, provide definitive results since normal subjects were used. However, there was a significant increase in total sleep, decrease in waking, and at least a tendency to a decrease in sleep latency when the drug was first given. Certainly, if an antidepressant is to be used and there are no clear indications for using another drug, amitriptyline would be indicated when insomnia is prominent.

However, the rebound increase in D-time and D-time percent, as well as the increases in fatigue and negative (usually groggy) feelings in the morning, not to mention the complex distortion of the usual interrelationships, makes one hesitate to recommend amitriptyline frequently for insomnia. It appears that in many ways the normal sleep patterns are distorted, and there is an especially prominent shift during the week after discontinuation.

This work was supported in part by National Institute of Mental Health Grant # MH 14520.

Bibliography

Akindele, M. O., Evans, J. I., Oswald, I.: Mono-amine oxidase inhibitors, sleep and mood. Electroenceph. clin. Neurophysiol. **29**, 47–56 (1970)

Allen, D. G., Bonica, J. J.: Amitriptyline (Elavil) as an agent for premedication. Anesthesiology **6**, 571–576 (1965)

Armstrong, R., Burnap, D., Jacobson, A., Kales, A., Ward, S., Golden, J.: Dreams and gastric secretions in duodenal ulcer patients. New Phys. **14**, 241–243 (1965)

Burt, C. G., Gordon, W. F., Holt, N. F., Hordern, A.: Amitriptyline in depressive states: A controlled trial. J. ment. Sci. **108**, 711–730 (1962)

Carlsson, A., Corrodi, H. Fuxe, K., Hokfelt, T.: Effect of antidepressant drugs on the depletion of intraneuronal brain 5-hydroxytryptamine stores caused by 4-methyl-alpha-ethyl-meta-tyramine. Europ. J. Pharmacol. **5**, 357–366 (1969 a)

Carlsson, A., Corrodi, H., Fuxe, K., Hokfelt, T.: Effects of some antidepressant drugs on the depletion of intraneuronal brain catecholamine stores caused by 4-alpha-dimethyl-meta-tyramine. Europ. J. Pharmacol. **5**, 367–373 (1969 b)

Coulter, J. B., Lester, B. K., Williams, H. L.: Reserpine and sleep. Psychopharmacologia (Berl.) **19**, 134–147 (1971)

Cramer, H., Kuhlo, W.: Effets des inhibiteurs de la monaminoxidase sure le sommeil et l'electroencephalogramme chez l'homme. Acta neurol. belg. **67**, 658–669 (1967)

Dobkin, A. B., Israel, J. S., Byles, P. H., Leep, P. K. Y.: Chlorprothixene and amitriptyline: Interaction with thiopentone. Circulatory effect and antisialogogue effect. Brit. J. Anaesth. **35**, 425–432 (1963)

Dunleavy, D. L. F., Brezinova, Y., Oswald, I., Maclean, A. W., Tinker, M.: Changes during weeks in effects of tricyclic drugs on the human sleeping brain. Brit. J. Psychiat. **120**, 663–672 (1972)

Glowinski, J., Axelrod, J.: Inhibition of uptake of tritiated noradrenaline in intact rat brain by imipramine and related compounds. Nature (Lond.) **204**, 1318–1319 (1964)

Greenberg, R., Pearlman, C.: Delerium tremens and dreaming. Amer. J. Psychiat. **124**, 133–142 (1967)

Gross, M. M., Goodenough, V. R.: Sleep disturbances in acute alcoholic psychoses. Psychiat. Res. Rep. Amer. Psychiat. Ass. **24**, 132–147 (1968)

Hartmann, E.: Reserpine: Its effect on the sleep-dream cycle in man. Psychopharmacologia (Berl.) **9**, 242–247 (1966)

Hartmann, E.: The effect of four drugs on sleep in man. Psychopharmacologia (Berl.) **12**, 346–353 (1968 a)

Hartmann, E.: Amitriptyline and imipramine: Effects on human sleep (Report to the Association for the Psychophysiological Study of Sleep, Denver, Colorado, March, 1968). Psychophysiology **5**, 207 (1968)

Hartmann, E.: Longitudinal studies of sleep and dream patterns in manic-depressive patients. Arch. gen. Psychiat. **19**, 312–329 (1968)

Hartmann, E., Baekeland, F., Zwilling, G., Hoy, P.: Sleep Need: How much sleep and what kind? Amer. J. Psychiat. **127**, 1001–1008 (1971)

Hartmann, E., Cravens, J.: The effects of long term administration of psychotropic drugs on human sleep: I. Methodology and the effects of placebo. Psychopharmacologia (Berl.) **33**, 153–167 (1973)

Himwich, H. E., Alpers, H. S.: Psychopharmacology. Ann. Rev. Pharmacol. **10**, 313–334 (1970)

Hoffmann, J. S., Domino, E. F.: Comparative effects of reserpine on the sleep cycle of man and cat. J. Pharmacol. exp. Ther. **170**, 190–198 (1969)

Hordern, A., Holt, N. F., Burt, C. G., Gordon, W. F.: Amitriptyline in depressive states. Phenomenology and prognostic considerations. Brit. J. Psychiat. **109**, 815–825 (1963)

Jouvet, M., Vimont, P., Delorme, F.: Suppression elective du sommeil paradoxal chez le chat par les inhibiteurs de la monoamineoxydase. C.R. Soc. Biol. (Paris) **159**, 1595–1599 (1965)

Khazan, N., Sawyer, C.: Mechanisms of paradoxial sleep as revealed by neurophysiologic and pharmacologic approaches in the rabbit. Psychopharmacologia (Berl.) **5**, 457–466 (1964)

Khazan, N., Sulman, F. G.: Effect of imipramine on paradoxical sleep in animals with reference to dreaming and enuresis. Psychopharmacologia (Berl.) **10**, 89–95 (1966)

Klerman, G. L., Cole, J. O.: Clinical pharmacology of imipramine and related antidepressant compounds. Pharmacol. Rev. **17**, 101–141 (1965)

Nowlin, J., Troyer, W., Jr., Collins, W., Silverman, G., Nichols, C., McIntosh, H., Estes, E., Bogdonoff, M.: The association of nocturnal angina pectoris with dreaming. Ann. intern. Med. **63**, 1040–1046 (1965)

Oswald, I.: Psychoactive drugs and sleep: Withdrawal rebound phenomena. Triangle **10**, 99–104 (1971)

Oswald, I., Brezinova, V., Dunleavy, D. L. F.: On the slowness of action of tricyclic antidepressant drugs. Brit. J. Psychiat. 120, 673–677 (1972)

Rosenblatt, G., Hartmann, E., Zwilling, G. R.: Cardiac irritability during sleep and dreaming. J. psychosom. Res. 17, 129 (1973)

Ryba, P., Engelhardt, D. M., Freedman, N., Shapiro, A.: The effects of imipramine on sleep patterns of psychiatric patients. Report to the Association for the psychophysiological study of sleep, Gainsville, Florida 1966

Schildkraut, J. J., Dodge, G. A., Logue, M. A.: Effects of tricyclic antidepressants on the uptake and metabolism of intracisternally administered norepinephrine-H^3 in rat brain. J. psychiat. Res. 7, 29–34 (1969)

Schildkraut, J. J., Draskoczy, P. R., Gershon, E. S., Reich, P., Grab, E. L.: Catecholamine metabolism in affective disorders. IV. Preliminary studies of norepinephrine metabolism in depressed patients treated with amitriptyline. J. psychiat. Res. 9, 173–185 (1972)

Schildkraut, J. J., Draskoczy, P. R., Gershon, E. S., Reich, P., Grab, E. L.: Effects of tricyclic antidepressants on norepinephrine metabolism: Basic and clinical studies. In: Brain chemistry and mental disease, Beng T. Ho and William M. McIssac (Eds.). New York: Plenum Publishing Corp. 1971

Stille, G.: Pharmacological investigation of antidepressant compounds. Pharmakopsychiat. Neuropsychopharm. 1, 92 (1968)

Urbach, K. F.: Hypnotic properties of amitriptyline: Comparison with secobarbital. Anesthesia and Analgesia. Curr. Res. 46, 835–842 (1967)

Vogel, G. W., Traub, A. C., Ben-Horin, P., Meyers, G. M.: REM deprivation. II. The effects on depressed patients. Arch. gen. Psychiat. 18, 301–311 (1968)

Wallach, M. B., Winters, W. D., Mandell, A. J., Spooner, C. E.: Effects of antidepressant drugs on wakefulness and sleep in the cat. Electroenceph. clin. Neurophysiol. 27, 574–580 (1969)

Wyatt, R. J., Fram, D. H., Kupfer, D. J., Snyder, F.: Total prolonged drug-induced REM sleep suppression in anxious-depressed patients. Arch. gen. Psychiat. 24, 145–155 (1971)

Wyatt, R. J., Kupfer, D. J., Scott, J., Robinson, D. S., Snyder, F.: Longitudinal studies of the effect of monoamine oxidase inhibitors on sleep in man. Psychopharmacologia (Berl.) 15, 236–244 (1969)

The Effects of Long-Term Administration of Psychotropic Drugs on Human Sleep: The Effects of Chlorpromazine

Ernest Hartmann and James Cravens

Sleep and Dream Laboratory, Boston State Hospital, Department of Psychiatry, Tufts University School of Medicine

Abstract. This paper reports on the effects of the daily administration of chlorpromazine (50 mg) to normal young males. Effects on laboratory recorded sleep, home sleep, and mood were studied.

Chlorpromazine significantly increased total sleep and decreased waking, especially on the first days, but to some extent throughout administration. Slow-wave sleep, D-time, and the stages of sleep considered individually were unchanged. Chlorpromazine had considerable effects on home sleep and mood variables. Some subjects clearly disliked chlorpromazine at this dose, and this was reflected by significant increases in the tension-anxiety, anger-hostility, and fatigue factors of the Psychiatric Out-patient Mood Scale (POMS). Overall what was most striking was the lack of effect on laboratory sleep measures in view of the effects on mood and home sleep reports.

Chlorpromazine (CPZ) is the most widely used major tranquilizer in the world today. Its clinical usage, almost always on a long-term basis, makes it imperative to determine effects such long-term administration may have on sleep patterns; the probable mechanisms of action of CPZ give such studies theoretical interest as well.

The exact action of chlorpromazine in the central nervous system is not known. It has a variety of effects on the nervous system, including shifts of the EEG to lower frequencies

(Fink, 1959, 1961), and a depressant action on the midbrain reticular activating system (Bradley, Wolstencroft, Hosli, and Avanizo, 1966) which could be related to its tranquilizing and antipsychotic properties. These effects do not clearly differentiate antipsychotic phenothiazines from those without antipsychotic potency. However, recent data suggest a specific mechanism of action—that chlorpromazine and the other antipsychotic phenothiazines may act in large as central dopamine receptor blockers (Nyback, 1971; Nyback, Borzecki and Sedvall, 1968; Matthysse (in press); Kety and Matthysse, 1972; Carlsson and Lindquist, 1963). The catecholamines are clearly implicated in the biochemistry of sleep and wakefulness (Jouvet, 1969; Hartmann, 1970, 1973), although the exact relationships are as yet uncertain. More specifically, animal studies suggest that the catecholamines, norepinephrine (NE) and dopamine (DA), may be necessary for maintaining normal wakefulness and it has been suggested that dopamine may be responsible for the behavioral signs of wakefulness (in the cat), whereas norepinephrine may have more to do with the EEG signs of wakefulness (Jones, Bobillier, and Jouvet, 1969). Here again long-term studies of chlorpromazine with observation of the effects on subjects' behavior and subjective as well as EEG recordings should be enlightening. We could consider the material from home reports, mood forms, etc., as somewhat analogous to observations of behavioral wakefulness in animals, though perhaps shedding more light on the details.

One of the early and consistent claims for CPZ has been that it tranquilizes without producing sleep or drowsiness, e.g., that it produces its clinical effect without disrupting normal wakefulness patterns. We can now examine this claim and in addition look at the dark side of life and ask whether CPZ produces its effects without disrupting normal sleep patterns.

There have been numerous studies of behavioral effects of CPZ, and a few studies of its sleep effects in animals (Hishikawa, Nakai, Ida and Kaneko, 1965; Khazan, and Sawyer, 1964; Jewett and Norton, 1966; Yamaguchi, Chikazawa, Ando,

Takeshima, and Takeuchi, 1971; Jouvet, 1967). In addition to the many findings of reduction of certain conditional responses, there are indications that at least in high dosage, chlorpromazine can increase sleep time and decrease desynchronized sleep (D) time.

There have been a number of studies on the effects of chlorpromazine and related phenothiazines on sleep in man, both in normal subjects and in psychiatric patients (Toyoda, 1964; Lester and Guerrero-Figueroa, 1966; Feinberg, Wender, Koresko, Gottlieb, and Piehuta, 1969; Lewis and Evans, 1969; Sagales, Erill, and Domino, 1969; Lester, Coulter, Cowden, and Williams, 1971; Ornstein, Whitman, Kramer, and Baldrige, 1969; Kupfer, Wyatt, Snyder, and Davis, 1971). The studies in normal subjects have all been single-dose or very short-term, with one exception (Lewis and Evans, 1969) which involved 3–7 nights of drug administration, while long-term studies on patients are somewhat difficult to evaluate. Table 1 summarizes studies to date of the effects of chlorpromazine on sleep in man, and includes the results of the present study for comparison.

Overall, the effect seems to depend somewhat on dosage, with low doses producing relatively little effect on initial administration, or perhaps a slight increase in sleep and D-time, whereas higher doses produce increased sleep and decreased D-time. Sleep latency is sometimes found to be reduced. There are certain conflicting results which the present long-term study may help to resolve. Our impression, based upon a number of unpublished studies and observations in psychiatric patients, suggests that there is definitely an interaction between direct effects on sleep and effects on mood or anxiety. Thus, within the tolerated dosage range, a normal person may have relatively little effect from CPZ, but there is no doubt that in an agitated patient or in some anxious subjects CPZ will greatly improve sleep, chiefly because of reduction of anxiety and agitation; such an improvement will be manifested as increased sleep time and also usually as decreased awakenings and increased D-time.

Table 1. Studies to date on the effects of chlorpromazine sleep in man

Author	Number of subjects	Type of subject	Length of time on drug	Dosage	Protocol design (nights in laboratory)	W-Time	Total sleep time
Toyoda, 1964	8	M and F, 5 normal, 3 patients (mixed dx)	Single dose	12.5 to 50 mg h.s.	No a; 1–3 bl; 1 d.		Slightly increased[1]
Lester and Guerrero-Figueroa, 1966	6	Normal M and F	Single dose	100 mg h.s.	1 a; 2 bl; 1 d; 1 ap (nc).	No change	No change
Feinberg et al., 1969	6	3M schizophrenics; 3M char. disorders	4–5 days	200 mg h.s.	5 bl; 4–5 d (c); 4–5 r.	No signif. change. Trend to decrease	No change
Lewis and Evans 1969 I.	4	Normal 2M, 2F	6–7 days	25 mg h.s.	1 a; 3–4 bl (nc); 5–6 d, 3 r (c).		Increase
II.	3	3M	3 days	100 mg h.s.	1 a; 3 bl (nc); 3d; 3 r (c).		
Sagales et al., 1969	8	Normal M	Single dose	0.4 mg/kg i.m.	1a; 1 bl; 1 d (nc)		
Lester et al., 1971	12	Normal M	Single dose	150 mg h.s.	1 a; 2 bl; 1 d; 1 r; 1 pbl (nc).	No change	No change
Kupfer et al., 1971 I.	5	M and F mixed psychiatric inpatients	3 or more days	100–300 mg/day	"several" a; 2 bl; "at least 3" d (c).	Decreased	Increased
II.	4	M and F mixed psychiatric inpatients	6–12 days	100 mg/day h.s. or divided.	"several" a; ? bl; 6–12 d.	Decreased	Increased
Hartmann and Cravens, 1973	10	Normal M	28 days	50 mg/day h.s.	2a; 3–4 bl. 8 d; 9 r; see text	Trend to decrease early	Increase early

a = adaptation; bl = baseline; d = drug; r = recovery; pbl = post-drug baseline; ap = additional placebo night at some point in the study between other drugs; c = consecutive; nc = nonconsecutive.
Blank spaces indicate data was either not obtained or not reported by authors.
[1] Exact data analyses and significance levels are not given in this study.

Table 1—continued

Author	Number of subjects	D-Time	S-Sleep Stages 1–4	Sleep latency	D-latency	S-D Cycle length	Number of body movements	Other findings
Toyoda, 1964	8	Increased[1]					Decreased at times	
Lester and Guerrero-Figueroa, 1966	6	No change	Increased Stage 4		No change			Increase is precentral fast (18–20/sec) activity
Feinberg et al., 1969	6	Decrease (% of sleep)	Increased Stage 4		No change		Decreased	No change in number of spindles. No change in EM density
Lewis and Evans 1969 I.	4	Increased (% of sleep)						No changes on recovery nights
II.	3		Decreased Stage 2	No change	No change			
Sagales et al., 1969	8	No change	Increased Stage 3; Decreased Stage 2		No change	No change	No change	No change in number of EMs
Lester et al., 1971	12	No change	Slight increase in SWS (stages 3–4)	No change	Reduced	No change	Reduced	Decrease in number of spindles during Stage 2. No change in EEG frequencies. No change in REM density
Kupfer et al., 1971 L	5	No change	No change in SWS	No change	No change	No change		REM density unchanged. Effect on sleep time diminishes over 6 days of administration
II.	4	No change	Increased Stage 2	No change	No change			Daytime chlorpromazine (100 mg/day) produced some of the changes at left, and was not distinguishable from placebo
Hartmann and Cravens, 1973	10	No change	No change	No change	No change	No change	Decrease	See text

[1] Exact data analyses and significance levels are not given in this study.

Legend for Tables

Laboratory variables:

Time Awake. All waking from start to end of EEG recording.

Number of Awakenings. Number of periods of awakening separated from other periods of waking by at least 5 min of sleep.

Sleep Latency. Time spent from start of recording until first Stage 1 which reaches

Stage 2.

Total Sleep Time. Sum of Stages 1, 2, 3, 4 and REM.

Stages 1, 2, 3 and 4: As defined in Rechtschaffen and Kales (1968).

Slow-Wave Sleep. Sum of Stages 3 and 4.

D-Time. Time spent in Stage REM.

D-Latency. Total time *asleep* before the first occurrence of Stage REM.

Number of D-Periods. Number of occurrences of Stage REM separated by more than 15 min.

Number of Stage Shifts. Total number of stage changes.

Cycle Length. Average time between ends of D-periods.

Number of Body Movements. Number of body movements more than 5 sec in length.

Disturbance Index. Sum of Number of Body Movements and Time Awake.

Home log variables:

Except for the *POMS* (Psychiatric Outpatient Mood Scale), home log variables are from daily responses in diaries kept by each subject. The POMS consists of an adjective checklist filled in weekly. Subjects were asked to consider their feeling for the entire week, not just that day.

For the present long-term study, a dose of 50 mg per night was chosen. Our preliminary studies suggested that, although by clinical standards 50 mg per day is a very low dose, it is also the highest dose that normal subjects can tolerate on a long-term basis. Thus there was little possibility for a dose-response curve study. In fact, our results (see below) strongly confirmed that we could not have used a larger dose.

METHODS

The methodology for this long-term study has been discussed in great detail in the first paper of this series (Hartmann and Cravens, 1973 a). Briefly, 14 subjects were studied for a total of 1,125 nights of recorded laboratory sleep. Subjects were normal males age 21–35. The design for each subject included six 60-day study periods, one for each of the following drug conditions, in a balanced design: placebo; reserpine 0.50 mg daily; amitriptyline 50 mg daily; chlorpromazine 50 mg daily; chloral hydrate 500 mg daily; and chlordiazepoxide 50 mg daily. Subjects, experimenters who ran studies at night, and assistants who scored the records were all blind as to drug condition.

During each 60-day period, the subject took a single pink capsule (drug or placebo) 20 min before bedtime every night for 28 nights, and then no medication for approximately 32 nights. Subjects slept in the laboratory the first five nights on medication, then once a week for the remainder of the medication period, then the first six nights after discontinuation of medication, then once a week for the remainder of the discontinuation period. The laboratory nights in a single study period would be approximately nights 1, 2, 3, 4, 5, 12, 18, 25, 29, 30, 31, 32, 33, 34, 42, 49, 55. In addition to these 17 nights of uninterrupted sleep each period includes one laboratory night during which the subject is awakened to study possible drug effect on dream content.

Subjects filled out a sleep log every morning throughout the study whether they slept at home or in the laboratory. They filled in time to bed, time up, estimate of time slept, any dreams, any unusual events or side effects, and then were asked to rate on a simple 5-point scale both the quality of their sleep for the night and how they felt that morning. Subjects filled out an adjective checklist—Psychiatric Outpatient Mood Scale (POMS)—once per week throughout the study, and were instructed to answer the questions for the entire past week, i.e., how they had tended to feel for that week, not how they were feeling at the time they filled out the form.

A total of ten subjects completed the two-month study period on CPZ, and of these, nine completed both CPZ and placebo periods. The statistical comparisons relating CPZ and placebo below refer to within-subject comparisons on the nine subjects who completed both conditions. Thus, for instance, a comparison of CPZ versus placebo for the first five days on medication involves obtaining the mean value for each variable on CPZ, and then the mean value on placebo for a given subject; measures of difference are then handled across subjects by *t*-tests for correlated samples.

RESULTS

The Effects of CPZ on Laboratory Sleep. Table 2 summarizes these results. In terms of overall sleep patterns there is a significant increase in total sleep when the medication is first given and concomitantly a trend toward decreased waking and number of awakenings (Fig. 1). The increased sleep is chiefly accounted for by an increase in stage 3. Total sleep time is still somewhat elevated on long-term administration of CPZ. For the eight study days through the month of administration, only one shows values below the placebo curve; this is day 4, when the values for placebo and CPZ are almost identical. Sleep time remains higher than placebo the first two days after discontinuation of medication (Fig. 2).

There is no significant change in total slow-wave sleep time (Fig. 3), or in stage 4 time separately, on medication, and no clear change after discontinuation. There is no significant change in total D-time (Fig. 4), D-percent, or D-latency, either immediately or on long-term administration; however, for the second through fourth weeks on medication, the number of D-periods is decreased and therefore the cycle length is increased. Body movements and stage shifts are slightly reduced.

Effect on Home Log Variables. On the whole, it is surprising how little effect CPZ had on major laboratory sleep variables. In contrast, CPZ had considerable effects on subjective and behavioral state (Table 3) as measured by morning sleep reports, POMS measures, and our impressions from the interviews. Subjects were often slightly groggy in the morning and occasionally noted a general tiredness or fatigue lasting through the day. On the POMS the *tension-anxiety*, the *anger-*

Table 2. Chlorpromazine: Effects on laboratory sleep

	On medication					Off medication				
	First night	First 3 nights	First 5 nights	Remaining nights	All nights	First night	First 3 nights	Second 3 nights	Remaining nights	Last night
Time awake (30-sec pages)	32.2 (−18.4)	34.2 (−19.4)	39.3 (−15.0)	37.1 (−3.5)	38.6 (−10.1)	47.9 (−4.0)	48.9 (+9.5)	40.8 (+5.9)	44.7 (+5.4)	42.4 (+6.9)
Number of awakenings	2.0	2.2	2.6	1.9	2.3	5.9	4.5	3.2	4.0	4.0
Sleep latency (30-sec pages)	21.1 (−5.2)	23.3 (−2.1)	24.8 (+1.1)	22.9 (+0.2)	24.2 (−1.2)	22.8 (−5.6)	25.4 (+5.5)	18.2 (−1.2)	22.4 (−2.4)	24.4 (+1.2)
Total sleep time (30-sec pages)	884 (+14.9)	888 (+28.9)	877 (+20.1)*	863 (+11.6)	871 (+15.6)	876 (+48.1)	870 (+26.3)	863 (+8.8)	859 (+17.0)	854 (+3.4)
Stage 1 (30-sec pages)	28.6 (−11.7)	34.9 (−3.5)	34.6 (−5.5)	27.8 (−8.8)*	32.2 (−6.8)	41.3 (+15.1)*	39.5 (+8.0)	38.5 (+7.4)	36.2 (+4.0)	32.8 (+3.6)
Stage 2 (30-sec pages)	462 (+47.6)*	450 (+16.7)*	446 (+13.5)	459 (+29.0)	450 (+17.7)	461 (+16.2)	455 (+0.7)	434 (+22.8)	443 (+7.8)	452 (+11.0)
Stage 3 (30-sec pages)	90.1 (−0.6)	92.5 (+19.3)*	89.4 (+18.3)***	72.4 (+0.1)	83.6 (+12.0)***	88.7 (+27.8)*	82.7 (+0.7)	69.1 (+7.7)	79.5 (−7.8)	69.1 (+0.8)
Stage 4 (30-sec pages)	87.9 (+4.7)	88.7 (−1.5)	87.5 (−4.1)	92.3 (+7.0)	89.9 (+0.9)	78.3 (−12.7)	74.1 (−10.4)	87.3 (−18.7)*	93.5 (−3.8)	105.3 (+8.7)
Slow-wave sleep (30-sec pages)	178 (+4.1)	181 (+17.8)	177 (+14.2)	165 (+7.1)	174 (+12.9)	167 (+15.1)	157 (+5.9)	156 (−11.0)	173 (+10.2)	174 (+9.4)
D-Time (30-sec pages)	215 (−25.1)	222 (−2.1)	219 (−2.1)	211 (−15.6)	215 (−8.2)	207 (−7.4)	219 (+11.7)	234 (−10.5)	206 (+10.6)	194 (−20.6)
D-Latency (30-sec pages)	164 (−9.4)	162 (−16.6)	164 (−12.5)	210 (+29.1)	180 (+2.8)	219 (+51.7)*	178 (+9.9)	162 (+21.4)	186 (+7.7)	192 (−9.6)
Number of D-periods	4.0 (−0.1)	4.2 (+0.1)	4.1 (+0.0)	3.6 (−0.6)***	3.9 (−0.2)***	4.3 (+0.3)	4.3 (+0.3)	4.4 (+0.1)	3.9 (−0.1)	3.8 (+0.0)
Number of stage shifts	57.4 (+1.9)	59.3 (+3.3)	58.3 (+2.0)	47.5 (+9.1)*	54.3 (−2.2)	63.8 (+12.2)*	60.9 (+6.8)	57.1 (+2.1)	60.1 (+3.5)	55.2 (−0.1)
Cycle length (30-sec pages)	229 (+17.3)	221 (+13.0)	218 (+0.4)	230 (+33.3)*	223 (+19.0)*	186 (−25.7)	204 (−9.9)	212 (+2.1)	211 (+2.6)	206 (−17.9)
Number of body movements	42.6 (−2.9)	41.9 (−7.2)	40.5 (−3.4)*	40.4 (−5.6)	40.5 (−7.4)*	50.2 (+4.8)	50.5 (+5.5)	50.3 (+5.1)	51.0 (+1.6)	51.2 (+4.1)
Disturbance index	74.8 (−21.3)	76.0 (−26.6)*	79.8 (−23.4)*	77.6 (−9.1)	79.1 (−17.5)*	98.1 (+0.8)	99.3 (+15.1)	91.0 (+11.0)	95.8 (+6.9)	93.7 (+11.0)

* $P < 0.05$; ** $P < 0.01$; *** $P < 0.001$. Numbers in parentheses indicate drug mean minus placebo mean.

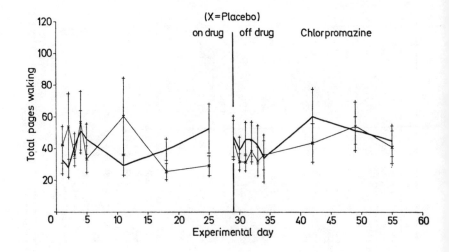

Fig. 1. Effects of chlorpromazine on time awake

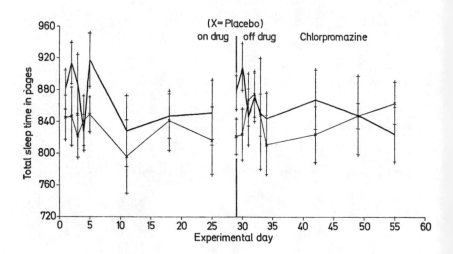

Fig. 2. Effects of chlorpromazine on total sleep time

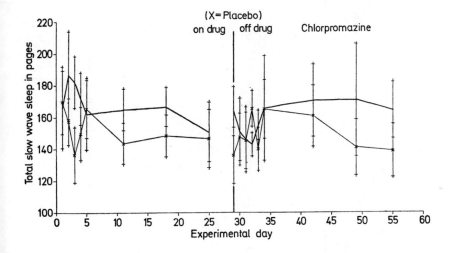

Fig. 3. Effects of chlorpromazine on slow wave sleep

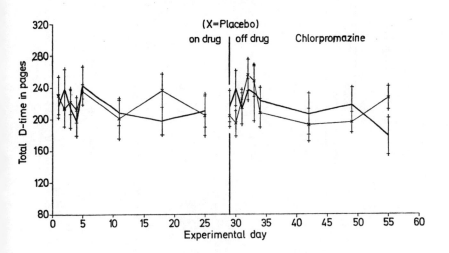

Fig. 4. Effects of chlorpromazine on D-time

Table 3. Chlorpromazine: Effects on home log variables

	On medication					Off medication				
	First week	Second week	Third week	Fourth week	All weeks	First week	Second week	Third week	Fourth week	All weeks
Estimated total sleep time (in hours and tenths)	7.4 (− 0.2)	6.9 (− 0.9)	6.7 (− 1.0)	7.0 (+ 0.2)	7.6 (− 0.1)	7.7 (+ 0.1)	7.9 (+ 0.3)	7.8 (+ 0.3)	6.6 (− 0.3)	7.6 (− 0.0)
Quality of sleep (1 = worst to 5 = best)	2.8 (− 0.1)	2.8 (− 0.2)	2.7 (− 0.3)	2.5 (− 0.1)	3.0 (+ 0.0)	2.8 (− 0.2)	3.0 (− 0.0)	3.0 (+ 0.1)	2.6 (− 0.2)*	2.9 (− 0.0)
How feel in the morning (1 = worst to 5 = best)	2.8 (− 0.1)	2.6 (− 0.4)	2.4 (− 0.6)	2.4 (− 0.2)	2.8 (− 0.1)*	2.9 (− 0.0)	2.9 (+ 0.1)	3.0 (+ 0.1)	2.5 (− 0.1)	2.9 (+ 0.0)
Feel sick in any way (mean number of positive responses)	0.3 (+ 0.0)	0.2 (+ 0.0)	0.2 (+ 0.1)	0.2 (+ 0.2)	0.2 (+ 0.0)	0.1 (+ 0.1)	0.1 (+ 0.1)	0.1 (+ 0.0)	0.1 (+ 0.0)	0.1 (+ 0.1)
Unusual psychological feelings (mean number of positive responses)	0.1 (+ 0.0)	0.1 (+ 0.1)	0.2 (+ 0.1)	0.2 (+ 0.2)	0.2 (+ 0.1)	0.1 (+ 0.0)	0.0 (− 0.1)	0.0 (− 0.1)	0.0 (− 0.0)	0.0 (− 0.0)
Fault of medication (mean number of positive responses — this refers to the two immediately preceding items and was only answered if there was a positive response to either)	0.2 (+ 0.0)	0.2 (+ 0.2)	0.2 (+ 0.2)	0.2 (+ 0.2)	0.2 (+ 0.0)	0.1 (+ 0.1)	0.0 (− 0.0)	0.0 (+ 0.0)	0.0 (+ 0.0)	0.1 (+ 0.0)

Table 3 (Continued)

Psychiatric Outpatient Mood Scale

Tension-anxiety	−0.1 (+1.3)	3.7 (+6.1)***	−0.2 (+1.4)*	−0.3 (+1.1)	1.1 (+2.9)**	−0.1 (+1.6)	0.1 (+1.2)*	−0.1 (+1.8)*	−0.1 (+1.5)	−0.2 (+1.0)*
Anger-hostility	−6.1 (+3.0)	−3.5 (+6.1)*	−4.0 (+5.2)	−4.1 (+4.2)	−5.3 (+4.0)	−4.0 (+3.7)	−6.1 (+1.6)	−7.6 (−0.8)	−8.3 (+2.1)	−6.4 (+0.5)
Fatigue	−2.3 (+2.2)	−0.6 (+3.6)**	−0.6 (+4.1)**	−1.4 (+2.6)	−1.5 (+3.0)**	−1.7 (+2.3)	−1.4 (+1.7)	−1.8 (+1.7)	−4.3 (−0.5)	−2.2 (+0.6)
Depression	−9.7 (−0.4)	−5.1 (+3.8)	−7.7 (+1.3)	−6.7 (+1.4)	−8.3 (+0.8)	−5.7 (+2.2)*	−6.2 (+1.3)*	−7.6 (+1.8)	−10.9 (−1.3)	−7.5 (+0.1)
Vigor	6.9 (−2.2)	5.1 (−2.2)	6.2 (−1.4)	5.0 (+1.2)	6.3 (−1.2)	5.9 (+0.4)	6.2 (−0.2)	6.7 (−0.2)	6.8 (−1.2)	6.7 (+0.2)
Confusion	1.0 (+0.7)	2.0 (+1.7)	0.5 (−0.6)	0.3 (−0.5)	1.1 (+0.4)	1.5 (+0.5)	1.1 (−0.1)	0.3 (+1.4)	−1.2 (+0.4)	0.5 (−0.4)

* $P < 0.05$; ** $P < 0.01$; *** $P < 0.001$. Numbers in parentheses indicate drug mean minus placebo mean.
For notes on Table 3, see page 000: "Home log variables."

hostility, and the *fatigue* factors all showed a significant increase at some period during CPZ administration, and scores tended to remain high for 1–2 weeks after drug discontinuation. The depression factor was not increased during administration of CPZ, but it rose significantly the first two weeks after discontinuation. CPZ produced more changes in the POMS than any other drug in these studies.

Although across subjects the number of complaints about side effects was not significantly increased, when the codes were broken it turned out that CPZ was the one condition under which two subjects had actually had some difficulty in continuing the study at the indicated dose.

Effect on Interrelationship. CPZ did not greatly affect the interrelationships between the laboratory variables found on placebo. (Amitriptyline was the only drug studied here which greatly altered these relationships.) CPZ did affect certain of the intercorrelations between laboratory sleep and mood or home log variables: For instance, quality of sleep versus waking time correlated − 0.34 on placebo, and + 0.10 on CPZ; POMS tension-anxiety versus waking time was + 0.34 on placebo, no relationship on CPZ. POMS fatigue versus sleep latency was − 0.42 on placebo, + 0.20 on CPZ. These changes are difficult to interpret but are consistent with the fact that CPZ produced relatively large changes in the POMS and relatively little change in laboratory sleep.

Discussion

Overall, CPZ had remarkably little effect on laboratory sleep variables, except for the initial increase in sleep. This study may perhaps help settle a long-standing controversy in the literature as to the effect of CPZ on D-time and D-time percent. We have found no alteration in D-time with the dosage employed here, which in our opinion is the largest dose tolerable on a continued basis by normal human subjects. Experience in our preliminary studies, as well as several studies in other laboratories on smaller dosages, make it likely that dosages lower than 50 mg also have essentially no effect on D-time in normal subjects. One study suggests that 25 mg may slightly increase D-time (Lewis and Evans, 1969) but the effect was not large and it is possible that a slow adaptation effect or a nonspecific antianxiety effect may have been involved.

It is still possible that very large doses of CPZ may produce an initial decrease in D-time (Feinberg et al., 1969), but this would not be remarkable since this is true of almost any medication; it may well be related to peripheral effects or side effects. The increased D-time sometimes reported after CPZ in mental patients (Kupfer et al., 1971) can most likely be attributed to a reduction of anxiety and the general amelioration of sleep.

It was striking that CPZ, despite its lack of influence on laboratory sleep patterns at 50 mg per day, produced definitely negative shifts in mood, as measured by the weekly POMS scale. This effect of CPZ in normal subjects has been noted previously, sometimes even on short-term or single-dose administration (DiMascio, Havens and Klerman, 1963 a, 1963 b). Thus DiMascio et al. in their correlations of drug activity and personality showed that one of their two personality types, Type A, characterized by a tendency to motor activity and extroversion, was also characterized by uncomfortable feelings on CPZ. The authors suggested that these subjects felt "tied down" or "doped" and unable to move in their usual way, and that this was very unpleasant to them. It is possible that our subjects reacted somewhat similarly.

However, in an attempt to verify this we correlated various personality measures (MMPI, etc.) with the percent of change from placebo caused by each drug. The results give no indication of any personality effect on the action of CPZ or the other drugs studied. However, with a small N (usually nine or ten) and a narrow range of scores on personality measurements across subjects, only a very marked effect would be detected.

The three instances noted in which CPZ produced clear

differences from placebo in intercorrelations make a certain amount of sense here. On placebo the relationships are expectable: subjects consider their sleep to be better, and report less anxiety, when their records show less waking time, and they have lower sleep latencies when they feel more fatigued. These relationships were all lost or reversed on CPZ, probably because of the large effects that CPZ itself had on the measures of mood.

The one significant effect found with CPZ on laboratory sleep variables—increase in total sleep—has been noted in other studies and may be of interest; it could be related to the probable dopamine receptor blocking actions of CPZ. In addition to a significant increase in laboratory sleep time in the first few days, total sleep remains slightly increased throughout the month of drug administration and the first days after. Taken in conjunction with the animal studies showing an increase in EEG sleep time on CPZ, usually at higher doses (Khazan and Sawyer, 1964; Jewett and Norton, 1966; Jouvet, 1967), one can conclude that one effect of this drug is to produce some increase in sleep at the expense of wakefulness, with no clear alteration in D-time. As mentioned, animal studies suggest a positive relationship between catecholamine activity and wakefulness; one study suggests a relationship between dopamine activity and *behavioral* (rather than EEG) wakefulness (Jones et al., 1969). We have found here significant, though small, effects of CPZ in reducing EEG wake fulness; in addition, the results we have discussed on the home log and mood measures could be seen as evidence of a possible reduction in "behavioral wakefulness." Thus the tiredness sometimes reported in the morning, the clear increase in "fatigue" and slight decrease in "vigor" on the POMS could relate directly to this effect, while the increase in "tension-anxiety" and particularly "anger-hostility" could be secondary effects of having to carry on normal life activities despite this "fatiguing" drug.

Also relevant here is a study just completed on the effects of pimozide on sleep in the rat (Hartmann, Zwilling, Koski and

List, 1973). Pimozide is an antipsychotic agent, related to the phenothiazines, which some studies have shown to have more clear-cut dopamine blocking properties that does CPZ. On pimozide at several dosages, we found a slight increase in sleep not quite reaching statistical significance, and absolutely no change in D-time. These results lend support to the view we have discussed that central dopamine activity is in some way necessary for wakefulness.

The lack of effect of these dopamine-receptor blockers on D-time may have important theoretical implications. We have shown in a number of animal and human studies that lowering catecholamine levels results in an increased D-time and increasing available catecholamines results in decreased D-time (Hartmann, Bridwell and Schildkraut, 1971; Hartmann and Chung, 1971; Hartmann, 1970). In fact, the effects of reserpine and amitriptyline demonstrated in this series of studies (Hartmann and Cravens, 1973 a, 1973 b) are consistent with these findings.[1] None of those drugs which alter catecholamine activity in the studies above can help us to differentiate between dopamine and norepinephrine. However, if central dopamine blocking (by CPZ and pimozide) produces no changes, it is likely that central norepinephrine rather than dopamine is involved in the effects on D-time.

We have suggested that there is a negative feedback system involving catecholamines and D-time such that reduced brain catecholamine levels, or "wearing out" of catecholamine systems, produces increased D-time which in turn results in restored catecholamine systems (Hartmann, 1970, 1973). The present results suggest that norepinephrine rather than dopamine systems are involved. Possibly the cortical and NE-dependent ascending systems (medial forebrain bundle, dorsal NE-bundle) responsible for attention, motivation, etc., gradually "wear out" during the day, so that by the end of

1. Reserpine, which acts by impeding storage of the biogenic amines, produces an increased D-time; amitriptyline, thought to act by making the amines more available at brain synapses, produces a decreased D-time.

the day there is relatively less synaptic activity or less efficient activity of these NE pathways. Sleep, and especially D-sleep, would then facilitate the restoration of NE levels or activity, returning them to functional integrity after the period of sleep. Drugs which reduce NE levels and increase D-time can be seen as producing an exaggeration or parody of what may happen during a normal wakeful day.

On a clinical level this study confirms the impression that CPZ can produce considerable mood changes chiefly in an unpleasant direction in normal subjects, and this should be kept in mind when the use of CPZ is considered, especially in an outpatient population.

However, the clearest finding here is that CPZ, in contrast with most medications studied, produces very little distortion of normal sleep patterns, and especially does not produce the reduction in D-time and in stage 4 so often produced by hypnotics and tranquilizers. This suggests that CPZ would not produce the many sleep problems, especially on discontinuation of medication, sometimes found after long-term use of sleeping medication, and thus suggests that CPZ may have some use as an occasional hypnotic in situations where anxiety is prominent.

This work was supported in part by National Institute of Mental Health Grant # MH 14520.

Bibliography

Bradley, P. B., Wostencroft, J. H., Hosli, L., Avanzino, G. L.: Neuronal basis for the central action of chlorpromazine. Nature (Lond.) **212**, 1425–1427 (1966)

Carlsson, A., Lindquist, M.: Effect of chlorpromazine or haloperidol on formation of 3-methoxytyramine and normatanephrine in mouse brain. Acta pharmacol. (Kbh.) **20**, 140–144 (1963).

DiMascio, A., Havens, L. L., Klerman, G. L.: I. Introduction, aims and methods. J. nerv. ment. Dis. **136**, 15–28 (1963)

DiMascio, A., Havens, L. L., Klerman, G. L.: The psychopharmacology of phenothiazine compounds. A comparative study of the effects of chlorpromazine promethazine, trifluoperazine and perphenazine in normal males. II. Results and Discussion. J. nerv. ment. Dis. **136**, 168–186 (1963)

Feinberg, I., Wender, P. H., Koresko, R. L., Gottlieb, F., Piehuta, J. A.: Differential effects of chlorpromazine and phenobarbital on EEG sleep patterns. J. Psychiat. Res. **7**, 101–109 (1969)

Fink, M.: Significance of EEG pattern changes in psychopharmacology. Electroenceph. clin. Neurophysiol. **11**, 391 (1959)

Fink, M.: Quantitative electronencephalography and human psychopharmacology. I. Frequency spectra and drug action. Med. exp. (Basel) **34**, 364–369 (1961)

Hartmann, E.: The D-state and norepinephrine dependent systems. In: Sleep and Dreaming, E. Hartmann (Ed.), pp. 308–328 Boston: Little, Brown 1970

Hartmann, E.: The functions of sleep. New Haven: Yale University Press 1973

Hartmann, E., Chung, R.: Effects of 6-hydroxydopamine on sleep in the rat. Nature (Lond.) **233**, 425–527 (1971)

Hartmann, E., Bridwell, T. J., Schildkraut, J. J.: Alpha-methylparatyrosine and sleep in the rat. Psychopharmacologia (Berl.) **21**, 157–164 (1961)

Hartmann, E., Cravens, J.: The effects of long-term administration of psychotropic drugs on human sleep: I. Methodology and the effects of placebo. Psychopharmacologia (Berl.) **33**, 153–167 (1973 a)

Hartmann, E., Cravens, J.: The effects of long-term administration of psychotropic drugs on human sleep: II. The effects of reserpine. Psychopharmacologia (Berl.) **33**, 169–184 (1973 b)

Hartmann, E., Cravens, J.: The effects of long-term administration of psychotropic drugs on human sleep: III. The effects of amitriptyline. Psychopharmacologia (Berl.) **33**, 185–202 (1973 c)

Hartmann, E., Zwilling, G., Koski, S., List, S.: The effects of pimozide on sleep in the rat. Report to the Association for the Psychophysiological Study of Sleep, San Diego, May 1973

Hishikawa, Y., Nakai, K., Ida, H., Kaneko, Z.: The effect of imipramine, desmethylimipramine and chlorpromazine on the sleep-wakefulness cycle of the cat. Electroenceph. clin. Neurophysiol. **19**, 518–521 (1965)

Jewett, R. E., Norton, S.: Effects of some stimulating and depressant drugs on sleep cycles of cats. Exp. Neurol. **15**, 463–474 (1966)

Jones, B. E., Bobillier, P., Jouvet, M.: Effets de la destruction des neurones cotenant des catecholamines du mesencephale sur le cycle veillesommeils du chat. C. R. Soc. Biol. (Paris) 163, 176–180 (1969)

Jouvet, M.: Mechanisms of the states of sleep: A neuropharmacological approach. Res. Publ. Ass. nerv. ment. Dis. 45, 86–126 (1967)

Jouvet, M.: Biogenic amines and the states of sleep. Science 163, 32 (1969)

Kety, S. S., Matthysse, S.: Prospects for research on schizophrenia: A report based on an NRP Work Session. Neurosci. Res. Progr. Bull. 10, 372–484 (1972)

Khazan, N., Sawyer, C. H.: Mechanism of paradoxical sleep as revealed by neurophysiologic and pharmacologic approaches in the rabbit. Psychopharmacologia (Berl.) 5, 457–466 (1964)

Kupfer, D. J., Wyatt, R. J., Snyder, F., Davis, J. M.: Chlorpromazine and sleep in psychiatric in psychiatric patients. Arch. gen. Psychiat. 24, 185–189 (1971)

Lester, B. K., Guerrero-Figueroa, R.: Effects of some drugs on electronencephalographic fast activity and dream time. Psychophysiology 2, 224–236 (1966)

Lester, B. K., Coulter, J. D., Cowden, L. C., Williams, H. L.: Chlorpromazine and human sleep. Psychopharmacologia (Berl.) 20, 280–287 (1971)

Lewis, S. A., Evans, J. I.: Dose effects of chlorpromazine on human sleep. Psychopharmacologia (Berl.) 14, 342–348 (1969)

Matthysse, S.: Schizophrenia: Relation to dopamine transmission, motor control, and feature extraction. Neurosciences third study program, Cambridge M.I.T. (in press)

Nyback, H., Borzecki, Z., Sedvall, G.: Accumulation and disappearance of catecholamines formed from tyrosine-^{14}C in mouse brain; effect of some psychotropic drugs. Europ. J. Pharmacol. 4, 395–403 (1968)

Nyback, H.: Effects of neuroleptic drugs on brain catecholamines neurons.: An experimental study using ^{14}C-labelled tyrosine. Karolinska Institut, Stockholm (thesis) (1971)

Ornstein, P. H., Whitman, R. M., Kramer, M., Baldridge, B. J.: Drugs and dreams IV. Tranquilizers and their effects upon dreams and dreaming in schizophrenic patients. Exp. Med. Surg. 27, 145–156 (1969)

Sagales, T., Erill, S., Domino, E. F.: Differential effects of scopolamine and chlorpromazine on REM and NREM sleep in normal male subjects. Clin. Pharmacol. Ther. 10, 522–529 (1969)

Toyoda, J.: The effects of chlorpromazine and imipramine on the human nocturnal sleep electroencephalogram. Folia psychiat. neurol. jap. 18, 198–221 (1964)

Yamaguchi, N., Chikazawa, S., Ando, J., Takeshima, T., Takeuchi, O.: The effect of psychotropic drugs on the sleep and levels of awareness in cats. Advance Neurol. Sci. (Tokyo) 14, 677–785 (1971)

The Effects of Long-Term Administration of Psychotropic Drugs on Human Sleep: The Effects of Chloral Hydrate

Ernest Hartmann and James Cravens

Sleep and Dream Laboratory, Boston State Hospital, Department of Psychiatry, Tufts University School of Medicine

Abstract. This paper reports on the effects of long-term administration of chloral hydrate (500 mg per day, at bedtime) on normal young males. The effects on laboratory sleep, home sleep, and mood were investigated.

Chloral hydrate significantly increased total sleep time and decreased sleep latency, even at the low dose used here. The effects were greater on the early days of administration. There was no effect on slow-wave sleep, D-time, or the stages of sleep studied separately. Chloral hydrate produced very little effect on mood or on subjective aspects of sleep, but it did produce distortion of the usual interrelationships between laboratory sleep and mood. Thus chloral hydrate, at 500 mg per night is definitely not a placebo. The paper discusses the differences between various currently used hypnotic agents.

Chloral hydrate (CH) is one of the oldest known hypnotic agents and is widely used throughout the world. It is thought to exert its actions through conversion to trichlorethanol which acts as a potent neural depressant, though the exact mechanism of action at a cellular level in the central nervous system is unknown (Marshall and Owens, 1954; Imboden and Lasagna, 1956; Goodman and Gilman, 1970). The effect of these substances on the complex mammalian nervous system is especially fascinating because of their chemical simplicity (Fig. 1). Chloral hydrate has been replaced to a certain extent by the more powerful barbiturates, but is still frequently used

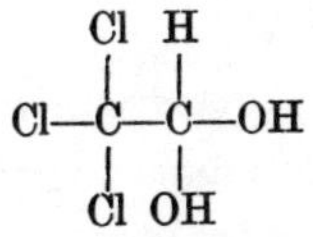

$$\text{Cl}\!-\!\overset{\overset{\displaystyle \text{Cl}}{|}}{\underset{\underset{\displaystyle \text{Cl}}{|}}{\text{C}}}\!-\!\overset{\overset{\displaystyle \text{H}}{|}}{\underset{\underset{\displaystyle \text{OH}}{|}}{\text{C}}}\!-\!\text{OH}$$

Fig. 1. Chloral hydrate

because it appears to produce fewer side effects as well as fewer problems on withdrawal compared to the barbiturates.

Short-term sleep EEG studies in several laboratories indicated that chloral hydrate might be a hypnotic which disturbs sleep patterning less than do the barbiturates; 500 mg or 1000 mg of CH at bedtime produced no suppression of desynchronized sleep time (D-time) (Kales, Jacobson, Kales, Marusak, and Hanley, 1968; Kales, Kales, Scharf, and Tan, 1970; Hartmann, unpubl.). Other stages of sleep were not greatly affected, and sleep latency in these normal subjects was reduced only at 1000 mg (Kales et al., 1970). In a longer study involving two weeks of nightly administration in four insomniac subjects, 1000 mg of CH tended to reduce sleep latency on the first few nights of administration, but latency returned to baseline levels after one to two weeks of continuous administration. Again, there was little change in the stages of sleep (Kales, Allen, Scharf, and Kales, 1970). There are no other published laboratory studies of long-term administration of CH in either normal or insomniac subjects.

A dose of 500 mg per night was chosen here because initial studies suggested that normal young subjects did not tolerate doses of 1000 mg per night continued over long periods; they frequently complained of grogginess in the morning.

Chloral hydrate is considered a relatively safe hypnotic, certainly in low doses such as used here, yet it is possible that repeated use of *any* hypnotic leads to some unpleasant effect such as mood changes during the day. And there are occasional reports of daytime problems after long-term administration. The present study, including daily home log forms and weekly mood scales, allows us to examine this question as well as the interrelationships of sleep and mood in a group of normal subjects.

The studies mentioned and authoritative sources (Goodman and Gilman, 1970) suggest that 500 mg of CH nightly has little pharmacologic effect on sleep patterns and may act chiefly as a placebo. This study should be able to detect this clearly by comparison of long-term administration of chloral hydrate and placebo within the same subjects. It will also be possible to compare, in the same subjects, the effects of CH, one of the oldest hypnotics, with the effects of chlordiazepoxide, chlorpromazine, and amitriptyline, all of which are sometimes used as hypnotic medication.

After presenting results on the long-term administration of CH, we shall compare it to other hypnotics and discuss more broadly the indications for and selection of hypnotic medication.

METHODS

The methodology for this long-term study has been discussed in great detail in the first paper of this series (Hartmann and Cravens, 1973 a). To summarize briefly, 14 subjects were studied for a total of 1,125 nights of recorded laboratory sleep. Subjects were normal males age 21–35. The design for each subject included six 60-day study periods, one for each of the following drug conditions, in a balanced design: placebo; reserpine 0.50 mg daily; amitriptyline 50 mg daily; chlorpromazine 50 mg daily; chloral hydrate 500 mg daily; and chlordiazepoxide 50 mg daily. Subjects, experimenters who ran studies at night, and assistants who scored the records were all blind to drug condition.

During each 60-day period, the subject took a single capsule (drug or placebo) 20 min before bed time every night for 28 nights, and then no medication for approximately 32 nights. Unfortunately, CH could not be packaged in a form exactly similar to the other medications; it was given as a clear red capsule without markings. Subjects slept in the laboratory the first five nights on medication, then once a week for the remainder of the medication period, then the first six nights after discontinuation of medication, then once a week for the remainder of the discontinuation period. The laboratory nights in a single study period would be approximately 1, 2, 3, 4, 5, 12, 18, 25, 29, 30, 31, 32, 33, 34, 42, 49, 55. In addition to these 17 nights of uninterrupted sleep, each period includes one laboratory night during which the subject is awakened to study possible drug effect on dream content.

Subjects filled out a sleep log every morning throughout the study whether they slept at home or in the laboratory. They filled in time to bed, time up, estimate of time slept, any dreams, any unusual events or side effects, and then were asked to rate on a simple 4-point scale both the quality of their sleep for the night and how they felt that morning. Subjects filled out an adjective checklist—Psychiatric Outpatient Mood Scale (POMS)—once per week throughout the study, and were instructed to answer the questions for the entire past week, i.e., how they had tended to feel for that week, not how they were feeling at the time they filled out the form.

A total of ten subjects completed the two-month study period on chloral hydrate, and of these, eight completed both chloral hydrate and placebo periods. The statistical comparisons relating chloral hydrate and placebo below refer to within-subject comparisons on the eight subjects who completed both drug conditions. Thus, for instance, a comparison of chloral hydrate versus placebo for the first five days on medication involves obtaining the mean value for each variable on chloral hydrate, and then the mean value on placebo for a given subject; measures of differences are then handled across subjects by t-tests for correlated samples.

RESULTS

Effects on Laboratory Sleep.
Overall results are presented in Table 1. There is no question that when first administered 500 mg of chloral hydrate alters sleep in the direction of an increase in total sleep time, a

Table 1. Chloral hydrate: Effects on laboratory sleep

	On medication					Off medication				
	First night	First 3 nights	First 5 nights	Remaining nights	All nights	First night	First 3 nights	Second 3 nights	Remaining nights	Last night
Time awake (30-sec pages)	27.2 (−26.5)	27.3 (−28.0)*	30.3 (−26.4)*	42.6 (+4.8)	34.6 (−14.5)	27.8 (−29.9)*	31.9 (−8.0)	42.7 (+8.5)	48.0 (+10.3)	26.6 (−9.1)
Number of awakenings	2.2 (−0.6)	2.3 (−0.9)	2.9 (−0.2)	3.9 (+1.6)	3.3 (+0.5)	1.1 (−1.9)***	2.2 (−1.1)	3.7 (+0.0)	3.4 (+0.5)	3.0 (+0.6)
Sleep latency (30-sec pages)	14.5 (−13.6)	15.3 (−9.6)*	13.8 (−9.6)	14.2 (−4.5)	13.9 (−7.5)	24.5 (−5.8)	18.7 (−0.7)	15.4 (−2.8)*	22.3 (−2.5)	15.8 (−6.9)
Total sleep time (30-sec pages)	881 (−12.2)*	867 (+22.1)	871 (+27.5)*	869 (+35.5)*	870 (+29.4)***	860 (+43.6)	862 (+36.2)*	843 (−3.8)	820 (−4.3)	804 (−21.6)
Stage 1 (30-sec pages)	29.2 (−6.2)	28.3 (−6.5)	33.4 (−3.2)	32.1 (−3.5)	32.9 (−3.5)	28.0 (+0.8)	26.8 (−2.4)	31.3 (+0.6)	32.3 (+3.0)	29.0 (+0.5)
Stage 2 (30-sec pages)	466 (+51.7)	488 (+58.0)*	468 (+41.6)*	457 (+38.8)	463 (+39.3)*	464 (+24.0)	457 (+16.1)	431 (−27.4)	417 (−25.8)*	381 (−45.4)
Stage 3 (30-sec pages)	83.9 (−13.6)	75.7 (−2.0)	73.6 (−2.8)	94.6 (+15.5)*	81.4 (+4.0)	78.9 (+13.9)	81.1 (+11.8)	72.4 (+5.4)	86.5 (+15.8)	102.5 (+27.6)
Stage 4 (30-sec pages)	77.4 (−8.0)	71.6 (−21.6)	84.4 (−7.4)	74.1 (−7.3)	81.1 (−6.6)	73.0 (−15.0)	79.1 (−1.5)	99.2 (−0.6)	84.2 (−8.7)	108.2 (+16.2)
Slow-wave Sleep (30-sec pages)	161 (−21.6)	147 (−23.6)	158 (−10.3)	169 (+8.2)	163 (−2.6)	152 (−1.1)	160 (+10.4)	172 (+4.8)	171 (+7.1)	211 (+43.9)
D-Time (30-sec pages)	224 (−2.6)	203 (−5.8)	212 (−0.7)	210 (−7.9)	211 (−3.7)	216 (+20.0)	218 (+12.1)	210 (−27.4)	200 (+11.4)	184 (−20.6)
D-Latency (30-sec pages)	252 (+76.6)*	204 (+20.6)*	189 (+7.4)	210 (+30.0)	197 (+17.2)	194 (+25.0)	170 (−1.0)	179 (+36.8)*	179 (−1.6)	184 (−27.9)
Number of D-periods	4.0 (−0.1)	4.2 (+0.2)	4.4 (+0.4)*	4.0 (−0.1)	4.3 (+0.2)	3.9 (−0.2)	4.1 (−0.0)	4.2 (−0.1)	3.8 (−0.0)	3.8 (+0.1)
Number of stage shifts	50.8 (−4.9)	48.8 (−6.7)	51.4 (−4.5)	58.5 (+1.3)	53.8 (−2.6)	55.8 (+1.6)	57.4 (+3.4)	58.6 (+1.1)	55.9 (−0.8)	54.5 (−1.9)
Cycle length	202 (−6.1)	199 (−5.9)	195 (−10.3)	200 (+4.8)	196 (−4.8)	210 (+10.4)	213 (+11.1)	194 (−9.1)	214 (+2.9)	202 (−23.2)
Number of body movements (30-sec pages)	42.1 (+0.2)	44.8 (−2.6)	44.8 (−2.7)	49.7 (+5.6)	46.5 (+0.4)	53.2 (+8.5)*	51.4 (+7.1)*	51.1 (+6.4)	46.2 (−1.8)	43.6 (−3.2)
Disturbance index	69.4 (−26.3)*	72.1 (−30.6)*	75.1 (−29.1)*	92.3 (+10.4)*	81.2 (−14.1)	81.0 (−21.4)	83.3 (−0.9)	93.8 (+14.9)	94.7 (+8.5)	70.2 (−12.4)

* $P < 0.05$; ** $P < 0.01$; *** $P < 0.001$. The numbers in parentheses indicate drug mean minus placebo mean.
For notes on Table 1, see page 000: "Laboratory variables."

decrease in waking time, and a decrease in sleep latency; there is some question as to how long these effects last. Thus total sleep time is significantly increased for the first five days on a drug, for the next three weeks on drug, for the entire period on drug taken together, and remains somewhat high on the first night after discontinuation. (Fig. 2).[1] The increased sleep is chiefly composed of stage 2 and occasionally stage 3. Waking time is significantly decreased for the first days on medication, shows no change for the remainder of time on medication, and a slight increase 5 to 6 days after discontinuation (Fig. 3). Sleep latency is significantly decreased for the first days on medication, still significantly decreased on day 12, but is no longer decreased by the third week on medication (day 18). There is no clear effect after this (Fig. 4).

Slow-wave sleep time and D-time are entirely unaffected by CH either during administration or after discontinuation (Figs. 5 and 6). In fact, the CH curve for slow-wave sleep is as close to placebo as any of the curves of this kind that we have seen. Fig. 6 (total D-time) and Fig. 7 (D-time percent) show the importance of determining long-term placebo curves and drug curves in the same subjects. If only the curves for chloral hydrate (heavy black lines) had been available, and comparisons made with a "baseline" period, one would have said that there was a definite "rebound" increase in D-time after discontinuation of the drug, most prominent on the third or fourth day after discontinuation. However, the increase on these days corresponded almost exactly with the increase found on placebo; thus there is no pharmacological effect.

D-latency, number of D-periods, and cycle lengths were not significantly affected by CH, though D-latency showed a trend toward an increase. The number of body movements and number of stage shifts showed no significant change

1. It appears that the second and fourth week on medication, sleep time is significantly longer on chloral hydrate than on placebo, the CH and placebo means are almost identical on the third week (Fig. 2); this may be merely a chance variation.

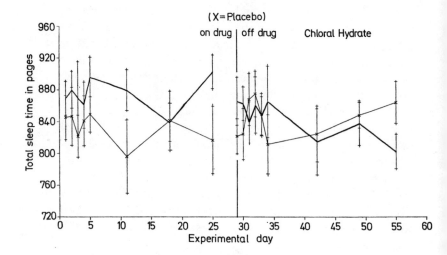

Fig. 2. Effect of chloral hydrate on total sleep

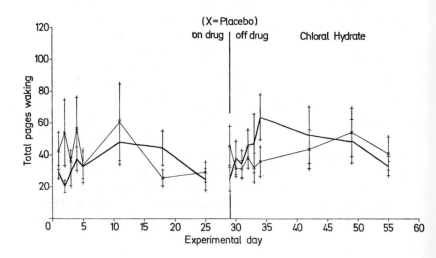

Fig. 3. Effect of chloral hydrate on waking time

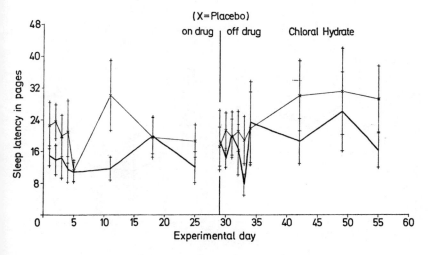

Fig. 4. Effect of chloral hydrate on sleep latency

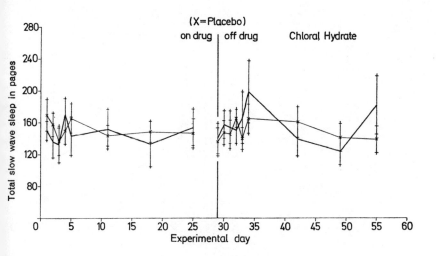

Fig. 5. Effect of chloral hydrate on slow-wave sleep

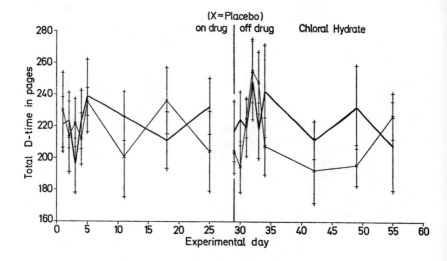

Fig. 6. Effect of chloral hydrate on D-time

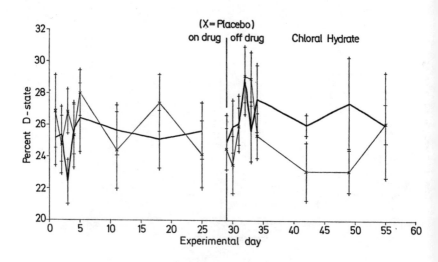

Fig. 7. Effect of chloral hydrate on D-time as a percent of total sleep

during drug administration, but the disturbance index (calculated by adding the number of body movements to the number of 30-second pages of waking after sleep onset) was significantly decreased for the first five days of CH administration.

On the whole, CH 500 mg per night produced increased sleep, decreased sleep latency and waking, and sleep disturbance, all most prominent for the first five nights, with relatively little shift in the internal organization of sleep.

Effect on Home Log Variables. Chloral hydrate produced no significant effect on how the subject felt in the morning or on his judgment of the quality of his sleep (Table 2).

There was little significant effect on the POMS mood scales; there was a trend during the first week of administration toward an increase in the tension-anxiety, fatigue, depression, and confusion factors; the confusion factor was increased for the entire drug administration period, but the amount of change was small. Overall, the number of significant differences from placebo in Table 2 is so small that it can very easily be due to chance alone. Thus CH had little or no effect on any subjective or mood variables.

Effects on Interrelationship. Chloral hydrate produced little change in the interrelationships between laboratory variables. However, it produced very large distortions of interrelationships between laboratory and home variables (Table 3). For instance, POMS vigor versus D-time showed 0 relationship on placebo but + 0.35 on chloral hydrate; POMS confusion versus D-time showed relationship at + 0.15 on placebo and − 0.42 on chloral hydrate; POMS depression versus sleep latency showed a relationship of + 0.25 on placebo and, similarly, values on the other drugs, but − 0.38 on chloral hydrate; POMS confusion versus sleep latency showed + 0.30 on placebo and most drugs but − 0.04 on chloral hydrate; POMS tension-anxiety versus disturbance index correlated + 0.20 on placebo and − 0.47 on chloral hydrate; POMS anger versus disturbance index showed relationships close to 0 for placebo and all drugs except for chloral hydrate on which there was a

Table 2. Chloral hydrate: Effects on home log variables

	On medication					Off medication				
	First week	Second week	Third week	Fourth week	All weeks	First week	Second week	Third week	Fourth week	All weeks
Estimated total sleep time (in hours and tenths)	7.6 (−0.1)	7.9 (−0.0)	7.9 (+0.2)	6.6 (+0.4)	7.8 (+0.1)	7.5 (+0.1)	8.0 (+0.4)*	6.5 (−1.2)	6.4 (−1.3)	7.7 (+0.2)
Quality of sleep (1 = worst to 5 = best)	3.1 (+0.1)	3.1 (+0.1)	3.0 (−0.1)	2.4 (−0.1)	3.0 (+0.0)	3.0 (+0.1)*	3.0 (−0.1)	2.4 (−0.6)	2.4 (−0.6)	2.9 (−0.0)
How feel in the morning (1 = worst to 5 = best)	2.8 (−0.1)	2.8 (−0.1)	2.9 (−0.1)	2.2 (−0.2)	2.8 (−0.1)	2.8 (−0.1)	3.0 (+0.1)*	2.4 (−0.5)	2.4 (−0.5)	2.8 (−0.0)
Feel sick in any way (mean number of positive responses)	0.1 (−0.1)*	0.1 (−0.2)	0.1 (−0.1)	0.0 (−0.0)	0.1 (−0.1)	0.0 (−0.1)	0.0 (+0.0)	0.1 (+0.1)	0.1 (−0.0)	0.0
Unusual psychological feelings (mean number of positive responses)	0.0 (−0.0)	0.1 (+0.0)	0.0 (−0.1)	0.0 (+0.0)	0.0 (−0.0)	0.0 (−0.1)	0.0 (−0.1)	0.0 (+0.1)	0.0 (−0.1)	0.0 (−0.1)
Fault of medication (mean number of positive responses—this refers to the two immediately preceding items and was only answered if there was a positive response to either)	0.0 (−0.2)	0.2 (+0.2)	0.0 (+0.0)	0.2 (+0.2)	0.2)+0.0)	0.0 (+0.0)	0.0 (+0.0)	0.0 (+0.0)	0.0 (+0.0)	0.0 (+0.0)
Psychiatric Outpatient Mood Scale:										
Tension-anxiety	0.4 (+2.2)	−1.2 (+1.4)	−2.3 (−0.2)	−2.3 (−0.6)	−1.7 (+0.5)	−1.2 (+1.1)	−1.8 (−0.2)	−3.2 (−1.8)	−2.9 (−0.7)	−1.7 (+0.2)
Anger-hostility	−7.5 (+1.8)	−7.7 (+1.8)	−7.7 (+1.1)	−8.2 (−1.2)	−8.8 (+0.3)	−9.1 (−0.9)	−9.5 (−1.5)	−9.0 (−2.6)	−8.6 (−3.2)	−9.2 (−2.4)
Fatigue	−1.8 (+3.0)	−3.8 (+0.8)	−3.4 (+2.0)	−1.8 (+2.6)	−3.1 (+1.9)	−4.4 (+1.5)	−4.6 (−0.0)	−3.4 (+0.2)	−3.6 (−0.3)	−4.4 (−0.2)
Depression	−7.4 (+5.2)	−12.2 (−1.2)	−10.0 (+0.6)	−9.5 (−0.7)	−10.6 (+0.6)	−11.1 (−1.2)	−11.2 (−2.0)	−11.9 (−2.4)	−10.9 (−1.0)	−11.1 (−1.4)
Vigor	6.0 (−3.4)	8.6 (+1.5)	8.4 (+0.8)	7.7 (+5.3)	8.1	7.6 (+1.7)	8.0 (+0.0)	6.7 (−1.6)	6.8 (−2.7)	7.9 (+0.0)
Confusion	1.1 (+2.5)	−0.9 (+0.5)	−1.2 (−0.4)	−0.8 (−0.5)	−0.3 (+0.7)	−0.2 (+0.8)	0.7 (+1.8)	−1.6 (−0.6)	−1.8 (−0.3)	0.1 (+1.3)

* $P < 0.05$; ** $P < 0.01$; *** $P < 0.005$. Numbers in parentheses indicate drug mean minus placebo mean.
For notes on Table 2, see page 000: "Home log variables."

Table 3. Correlations between laboratory and mood (POMS) variables

	Tension-anxiety		Anger-hostility		Fatigue		Depression		Vigor		Confusion	
Time awake	−0.13 (0.06)	0.30	−0.31 (0.04)	−0.29	−0.08 (0.15)	0.01	−0.28 (0.05)	−0.14	0.06 (−0.03)	0.07	−0.19 (0.10)	−0.05
Sleep latency	0.10 (0.14)	0.28	−0.40 (−0.01)	0.07	0.08 (0.14)	0.42	−0.38 (0.11)	0.25	0.02 (−0.15)	−0.09	−0.04 (0.26)	0.32
Disturbance index	−0.47 (−0.06)	0.22	−0.33 (−0.04)	0.11	−0.51 (0.11)	0.30	−0.30 (−0.01)	0.24	−0.13 (−0.05)	−0.08	−0.48 (0.06)	0.26
Total sleep time	−0.39 (0.06)	0.05	0.11 (0.10)	0.06	−0.26 (0.08)	−0.03	0.15 (0.13)	0.11	0.02 (−0.11)	0.15	−0.17 (0.15)	0.14
Slow-wave sleep	−0.08 (−0.03)	−0.23	0.50 (0.14)	0.01	0.21 (−0.05)	−0.39	0.32 (−0.05)	−0.19	−0.28 (0.07)	0.16	0.02 (−0.13)	−0.30
D-Time	−0.55 (−0.04)	−0.05	−0.25 (−0.06)	−0.16	−0.58 (−0.05)	−0.04	−0.17 (0.09)	0.05	0.35 (−0.11)	0.04	−0.42 (0.18)	0.15

Correlations between laboratory and mood (POMS) variables. In each cell are presented above center for all nights on chloral hydrate; below left in parentheses for all nights in entire study; and below right for all nights on placebo. i.e.::

$$r_{ch}$$
$$(r_{total})\ r_{placebo}$$

correlation of − 0.30; POMS fatigue versus disturbance index showed a relationship of + 0.30 on placebo and − 0.50 on chloral hydrate; POMS fatigue versus slow-wave sleep related − 0.40 on placebo and + 0.20 chloral hydrate; POMS depression versus disturbance index + 0.24 on placebo and − 0.30 on chloral hydrate; and finally, POMS confusion versus disturbance index + 0.26 on placebo and − 0.48 on chloral hydrate.

It is difficult to interpret each of the specific correlations, but clearly CH produced a profound disruption of normal interrelationships between laboratory variables and the subjects' home log and mood variables. A great many of the relationships were actually *reversed* on CH and the differences from placebo were highly significant.

CONCLUSIONS AND DISCUSSION

Even in the low dose employed here, and in normal, noninsomniac subjects, where there was little room for "improved" sleep, CH had a hypnotic effect, i.e., it increased total sleep, decreased waking and decreased sleep latency for the first days of administration. Thus CH 500 mg per night is not a placebo. As mentioned, data for the later weeks on medication are somewhat harder to interpret, and show less clear-cut effects on sleep, though total sleep is still significantly increased. It is somewhat surprising that 500 mg of CH produced significant decreases in sleep latency in these subjects and not in the normal subjects studied by Kales et al. (1970). Our subjects who showed a mean sleep latency of only 11 min on placebo were not ideal ones in whom to find a reduced latency. On the other hand, our subjects were very reliable, had stable sleep patterns, and were unusually well adapted to the laboratory; thus, the intrasubject variation in sleep latency was quite low; this low variability helps make small differences statistically significant.

Aside from the above changes, CH produced little disturbance in laboratory sleep organization and little or no effect on subjective reports. In view of these negative findings, the changes produced in the interrelationships between laboratory and home log variables are especially striking. No simple explanation comes to mind to account for the specific altered relationships. It does seem that the normal relationships between a person's subjective feelings and his brain activity, as measured by sleeping EEG, are somehow disrupted while he is under the influence of CH. This may be related to the mild feelings of strangeness and discomfort felt by some persons taking hypnotics, though such feelings were not prominent here. Small changes in the direction of feeling unusual or "worse" just when EEG sleep looked "better" could have a large effect on the interrelations.

These results suggest that whatever effect on mood and home estimates is being produced, it is perhaps produced in a different way by CH than by the other medications used in this study. Chlordiazepoxide was found to produce little effect on the home log variables and little change in the interrelationships (Hartmann and Cravens, 1973 e). Reserpine, amitriptyline, and chlorpromazine all produced a variety of changes on the home variables but produced relatively little change in the interrelationships (Hartmann and Cravens, 1973 b, 1973 c, 1973 d). In other words, for these drugs, even when changes in mood and experience were produced, relationships between these changes and brain function as measured by sleep EEG were not greatly altered. Possibly the three medications, reserpine, amitriptyline, and chlorpromazine, all of which probably act on CNS catecholamine systems, may alter brain systems in a way that is somehow familiar to the subject, i.e., the way they may normally be altered at times of activation and high energy or at times of fatigue, at times of happiness or sadness. CH could be seen as acting in some clearly different way so that the usual interrelationships are distorted.

In trying to compare CH with other drugs used in this study, the first point is that CH had a hypnotic effect but produced little change or distortion of sleep laboratory variables such as sleep stages or cycling. The other drugs studied produced greater changes, except for chlorpromazine. The increase in sleep time on the first day of CH is similar to the increases found with chlorpromazine and with amitriptyline, but only CH produced a significant decrease in sleep latency. It is to be noted that none of these drugs had a clearly significant effect on total sleep or sleep latency after 3 to 4 weeks of administration.

It is important also to compare chloral hydrate with other hypnotics in widespread use. The barbiturates, of course, are the other group of old and widely used hypnotics; these have been studied many times in the sleep laboratory (see Freemon, 1972; King, 1972; Hartmann, 1970; for reviews). Studies of single-dose administration of clinical doses of barbiturates (for instance, 100 mg of pentobarbital or seconal) show slightly increased total sleep time and decreased sleep latency. D-time is reduced and D-latency increased. Kales et al. (1970), studying several nights of administration of 100 mg of pentobarbital followed by withdrawal in a small number of subjects, found no significant reduction in waking time or sleep latency but a decrease in stage 4 sleep and D-time during administration and an increase in D-time on withdrawal. It seems clear that on short-term administration, CH in clinical dosage can produce hypnotic effects similar to those of the usual clinical dose of pentobarbital, without the alteration in sleep stages produced by the barbiturates.

It has been suggested that flurazepam has superior hypnotic properties to CH and maintains its effect in reducing sleep latency for a number of weeks. We have previously studied flurazepam (30 mg) as well as chlordiazepoxide (100 mg) on single nights (1968); both drugs did produce significantly reduced sleep latency and increased sleep somewhat, as we found in the study of CH. On long-term administration, we found no increased sleep or reduced sleep latency on 50 mg of chlordiazepoxide (Librium), a benzodiazepine closely related to flurazepam (1973 e), although reduced latency has been reported after 30 mg of flurazepam given for two weeks to insomniacs (Kales et al., 1970). Our present study of chlordiazepoxide, as well as several studies in other laboratories (Kales et al., 1970; Oswald and Priest, 1965) also suggest that benzodiazepines produce considerable changes in sleep patterns—definite reductions in D-time and in slow-wave sleep on continuous administration—which were not produced by CH. It can be considered an advantage in the use of CH that there is not a great decrease in these variables, and no "rebound" increase on discontinuation. Thus the period of distress, sometimes accompanied by poor sleep and nightmares, so frequently reported after withdrawal of barbiturates, appears not to occur after CH.

A number of other hypnotic drugs have been studied in and out of the sleep laboratory (Freemon, 1972). A complete review is not indicated here, but our impression of the data is that none of these has been shown to have effects superior to those of CH or flurazepam.

This study again demonstrates that the body develops tolerance to the sleep time and sleep latency effects. A normal subject who has taken CH continuously for 2 to 4 weeks shows laboratory sleep stages almost indistinguishable from his sleep on placebo. Pharmacologically this is not especially surprising; it suggests that the systems in the brain involved in regulating sleep and waking are, like many other neural systems, under the control of sensitive negative feedback mechanisms. Clinically, this raises the serious question of whether any hypnotic is useful on a long-term basis, or whether a hypnotic should be prescribed only on a short-term basis for transient difficulties with sleep. Obviously there is a great deal to be said for the latter position.

Our impression is that, at least in younger age groups, insomnia is usually a sleep-onset insomnia most commonly related to anxiety. Frequently the relief of anxiety by psychotherapy or similar techniques, or a simple alteration of the patient's environment or habits can produce a great improvement in insomia. It is also noteworthy that not all persons with long sleep latencies seek medical help for insomnia. That is, some persons regularly encounter problems falling asleep, but get up and read, study, work around the house, etc., until they are able to sleep and hardly seem to be anxious about or incapacitated by insomnia.

Possibly some insomniacs, especially older ones, may have a "primary" or "essential" insomnia in the sense of insufficiency of a chemical substrate or enzyme, or lowered permeability of a membrane to some substance, etc. At this stage in our knowledge we might guess that insufficient availability or turnover of serotonin could be involved. In such cases, a drug increasing the availability of serotonin might be indicated, and we have shown that l-tryptophan reduces sleep latency without altering sleep stages in animals (Hartmann and Chung, 1972), in normal subjects (Hartmann, Chung, and Chien, 1971), and in insomniacs (Hartmann, 1973).

In our opinion, the immediate prescription of a sleeping pill to be taken on a long-term basis is seldom indicated. Rather, the insomniac should first have a careful medical and psychiatric work-up; if no medical illness accounting for the insomnia is found (and there are many such possibilities), the possible reasons for anxiety, especially the fear of letting go, can be explored psychiatrically. If psychotherapy is not possible or acceptable, many simple measures such as modifying diet or life patterns can be helpful. If none of these is effective, a substance such as l-tryptophan or one of the standard hypnotics could be considered on a short-term basis. Thus, chloral hydrate and other hypnotics are left with a somewhat limited role as agents to be used transiently in situational insomnias, or again transiently while a more long-term and specific treatment is being sought.

This work was supported in part by National Institute of Mental Health Grant # MH 14520.

Bibliography

Freemon, F. R.: Sleep Research: A critical review. Springfield, Ill.: Ch. C. Thomas 1972
Goodman, L. S., Gilman, A.: The pharmacological basis of therapeutics. Fourth edition. London-Toronto: Macmillan Comp. 1970

Hartmann, E.: The effect of four drugs on sleep in man. Psychopharmacologia (Berl.) **12**, 346–353 (1968)

Hartmann, E.: Pharmacological studies of sleep and dreaming: Chemical and clinical relationships. Biol. Psychiat. **1**, 243–258 (1970)

Hartmann, E., Chung, R.: Sleep inducing effects of l-tryptophane. J. Pharm. Pharmacol. **24**, 252–253 (1972)

Hartmann, E., Chung, R., Chien, C.: l-Tryptophane and sleep. Psychopharmacologia (Berl.) **19**, 114–127 (1971)

Hartmann, E., Cravens, J.: The effects of long-term administration of psychotropic drungs on human sleep, I. Methodology and the effects of placebo. Psychopharmacologia (Berl.) **33**, 153–167 (1973 a)

Hartmann, E., Cravens, J.: The effects of long-term administration of psychotropic drugs on human sleep. II. The effects of reserpine. Psychopharmacologia (Berl.) **33**, 169–184 (1973 b)

Hartmann, E., Cravens, J.: The effects of long-term administration of psychotropic drugs on human sleep. III. The effects of amitriptyline. Psychopharmacologia (Berl.) **33**, 185–202 (1973 c)

Hartmann, E., Cravens, J.: The effects of long-term administration of psychotropic drugs on human sleep. IV. The effects of chlorpromazine. Psychopharmacologia (Berl.) **33**, 203–218 (1973 d)

Hartmann, E., Cravens, J.: The effects of long-term administration of psychotropic drugs on human sleep. VI. The effects of chlordiazepoxide. Psychopharmacologia (Berl.) **33**, 233–245 (1973 e)

Imboden, J., Lasagna, L.: An evaluation of hypnotic drugs in psychiatric patients. Bull. Johns Hopk. Hosp. **99**, 1–100 (1956)

Kales, A., Allen, C., Scharf, M. B., Kales, J. D.: Hypnotic drugs and their effectiveness. All-night EEG studies of insomniac subjects. Arch. Gen. Psychiat. **23**, 226–232 (1970)

Kales, A., Jacobson, A., Kales, J. D., Marusak, C., Hanley, J.: Effects of drugs on sleep (Noludar, Doriden, Nembutal, Chloral hydrate, Benadryl). Psychophysiology **4**, 391–392 (Abs.) (1968)

Kales, A., Kales, J. D.: Sleep laboratory evaluation of psychoactive drugs. Pharmacol. Physcns. **4**, 1–6 (1970)

Kales, A., Kales, J. D., Scharf, M. B., Tan, T-L: Hypnotics and altered sleep-dream patterns. 2. All-night EEG studies of chloral hydrate, flurazepam, and methaqualone. Arch. Gen. Psychiat. **23**, 219–225 (1970)

Kales, A., Preston, T. A., Tan, T.-L., Allen, C.: Hypnotics and altered sleep-dream patterns. 1. All-night EEG studies of flutethimide, methyprylon, and pentobarbital. Arch. Gen. Psychiat. **23**, 211–218 (1970)

King, C. D.: The pharmacology of rapid eye movement sleep. Advanc. Pharmacol. Chemother. **9**, 1 (Monogr.) (1972)

Marshall, E. K., Jr., Owens, A. H., Jr.: Absorption, excretion and metabolic rate of chloral hydrate and trichloroethanol. Bull. Johns Hopk. Hosp. **95**, 1–18 (1954)

Oswald, I., Priest, R. G.: Five weeks to escape the sleeping pill habit. Brit. Med. J. **1965**II, 1093–1099

The Effects of Long-Term Administration of Psychotropic Drugs on Human Sleep: The Effects of Chlordiazepoxide

Ernest Hartmann and James Cravens

Sleep and Dream Laboratory, Boston State Hospital, Department of Psychiatry, Tufts University School of Medicine

Abstract. This paper reports on the effects of long-term administration of chlordiazepoxide (CDX) (50 mg per day at bedtime) on normal young males. The effects on laboratory sleep, home sleep, and mood were investigated.

CDX produced an immediate increase in sleep time, but this returned to placebo levels after 2–3 days. Slow-wave sleep (stages 3 and 4) was normal for the first few days, but then showed a great decrease and remained significantly low throughout the period of drug administration, and for the first week after discontinuation. D-time similarly is not greatly affected for the first days, but is then decreased for the remainder of the four weeks on medication. During the period when both slow-wave sleep and D-time are decreased, stage 2 sleep is greatly increased. CDX produced little effect on mood; subjective "quality of sleep" was judged better on CDX than on placebo by these subjects.

Chlordiazepoxide (CDX), one of the benzodiazepines, was introduced into clinical use in 1961 and is probably the most widely used minor tranquilizer in the United States today and one of the most widely used drugs of any category. Some physicians prescribe CDX (Librium®) in small doses for a great variety of conditions that are or could be accompanied by stress or anxiety. The impression appears to be that a small dose of Librium won't do any harm and may help a bit whether the effect is pharmacological or chiefly a placebo effect. The antianxiety effects of CDX have been widely studied with generally positive results (Randall, 1961; Goodman and Hilman, 1970; Rickels, 1968). The effects on sleep have not been adequately studied.

The mechanisms by which CDX and the other benzodiazepines reduce anxiety are not clearly understood. These drugs reduce aggression in animals (Randall, 1961), have general sedative and anticonvulsive effects, and large doses produce general slowing of the waking EEG in man (Randall, 1961; Goodman and Gilman, 1970). All these could be related to antianxiety effects, but all are nonspecific, and can be produced by agents that have no clinical antianxiety effects. These effects may be secondary to alteration of electrical activity in the reticular activating system, including depression of spinal reflex activity and reduction of spontaneous discharge rates in some reticular activating system neurons (Przybyla and Wang, 1968). A recent more specific neurochemical suggestion is that the benzodiazepines may exert an antianxiety effect by reducing brain serotonin turnover (Wise, Berger, and Stein, 1972), since the time-course of increased appearance of punishment-suppressed behavior in the rat is very similar to the time-course of decreased serotonin turnover (but not turnover of other amines) after benzodiazepine administration.

CDX is thought to be an extremely safe medication, with a high therapeutic index, and with few side effects on long-term administration. This study, involving sleep EEG variables as well as daily subjective reports, allows us to examine effects of CDX quantitatively over time in a normal population.

Short-term studies at first indicated that CDX and related benzodiazepines produced little effect on sleep. One study in our laboratory involved ten subjects who took placebo, pentobarbital, amitriptyline, CDX, and another benzodiazepine—flurazepam—in a crossover design (Hartmann, 1968). Single bedtime doses of CDX (100 mg) or flurazepam (30 mg) produced a significant increase in total sleep with no other obvious changes; there was a trend toward decreased sleep latency, decreased D-time, and decreased stages 3 and 4 sleep which did not reach significance. It has been shown that flurazepam, administered for 14 days, produces a significant reduction in slow-wave sleep (stage 3 and 4 sleep) (Kales, Kales, Scharf, and Tan, 1970). The same effects appear to occur with other benzodiazepines less methodically studied (Monti, Trenchi, and Morales, 1971; Haider and Oswald, 1971; Erhart, 1971). This may have detrimental aspects, but it may also make these drugs useful for treatment of such conditions as nightmares, sleep walking, and other sleep disorders which arise from stage 4 of sleep. Several studies have already investigated such uses (Glick, Schulman, and Turecki, 1971; Erhart, 1971). Diazepam (Valium) given in low doses has been found to be quite useful in treating patients with stage 4 nightmares (Fisher, Byrne, Edwards, and Kahn, 1970).

CDX is also of interest because although it is officially sold as a tranquilizer, physicians often recommend it as a nighttime hypnotic as well, and some recent related benzodiazepines, especially flurazepam, have been marketed specifically as hypnotics.

A long-term study in insomniac patients indicated that 30 mg of flurazepam greatly reduced sleep latency and slightly increased sleep time in insomniac patients during the entire two weeks of administration. In these patients a marked decrease in stage 4 was noted (Kales, Allen, Scharf, and Kales, 1970; Kales, Kales, Bixler, and Slyde, 1971).

In all these drug studies we are also interested in whether the medication will produce its clinical effects when used in low dosage in normal subjects. With CDX, the question is whether there will be a tranquilizing effect or some effect on mood, and whether this will be related to the sleep effects.

The present study allows us to compare this widely used medication with other tranquilizers and other hypnotics as well as with placebo in the same normal subject group. Since these subjects are neither insomniac nor particularly anxious, this is not a group in which effects in reducing anxiety or on inducing sleep can be very easily noted. However, because of the stability of the subjects and the low variation on most measures, it was a good group in which we could look for any possible disruptions or other effects on sleep produced by long-term use.

METHODS

The methodology for this long-term study has been discussed in great detail in the first paper of this series (Hartmann and Cravens, 1973 a). Briefly, 14 subjects were studied for a total of 1,125 nights of recorded laboratory sleep. Subjects were normal males age 21–35. The design for each subject included six 60-day study periods, one for each of the following drug conditions, in a balanced design: placebo; reserpine 0.50 mg daily; amitriptyline 50 mg daily; chlorpromazine 50 mg daily; chloral hydrate 500 mg daily; and chlordiazepoxide 50 mg daily. Subjects, experimenters who ran studies at night, and assistants who scored the records were all blind to drug condition.

During each 60-day period, the subject took a single pink capsule (drug or placebo) 20 min before bedtime every night for 28 nights, and then no medication for approximately 32 nights. Subjects slept in the laboratory the first five nights on medication, then once a week for the remainder of the medication period, then the first six nights after discontinuation of medication, then once a week for the remainder of the discontinuation period. The laboratory nights in a single study period would usually be nights 1, 2, 3, 4, 5, 12, 18, 25, 29, 30, 31, 32, 33, 34, 42, 49, 55. In addition to these 17 nights of uninterrupted sleep, each period includes one laboratory night during which the subject is awakened to study possible drug effect on dream content.

Subjects filled out a sleep log every morning throughout the study whether they slept at home or in the laboratory. They filled in time to bed, time up, estimate of time slept, any dreams, any unusual events or side effects, and then were asked to rate on a simple 5-point scale both the quality of their sleep for the night and how they felt that morning. Subjects filled out an adjective checklist—Psychiatric Outpatient Mood Scale (POMS)—once per week throughout the study, and were instructed to answer the questions for the entire past week, i.e., how they had tended to feel for that week, not how they were feeling at the time they filled out the form.

A total of 9 subjects completed the two-month study period on CDX, and of these, 8 completed both CDX and placebo periods. The statistical comparison relating CDX and placebo below refer to within-subject comparisons on the 8 subjects who completed both drug conditions. Thus, for instance, a comparison of CDX versus placebo for the first five days on medication involves obtaining the mean value for each variable on CDX, and then the mean value on placebo for a given subject; measures of difference are then handled across subjects by *t*-tests for correlated samples.

RESULTS

The Effects of CDX on Laboratory Sleep. The results are summarized in Table 1. CDX produces an immediate significant increase in total sleep time (Fig. 1) with a decrease in waking and a trend toward reduced sleep latency. However, after the first three days, total sleep time is not differentiable from placebo and the same is true of total waking time and sleep latency. Slow-wave sleep (Fig. 2) and also stage 4 taken separately (Table 1), show a decrease significant during the first days of administration, and an even larger decrease thereafter, so that there is a very significant reduction in slow-wave sleep for the entire month on medication. The reduction in slow-wave sleep continues through at least the first week after discontinuation of medication and does not reach placebo levels until the second week off drug. This effect is surprisingly clear-cut: There is no cross-over of the placebo time-curve and the CDX time-curve until day 42 of the study (Fig. 2). There is no indication of a "rebound." Stage 2 sleep is significantly increased throughout

Table 1. Chlordiazepoxide: Effects on laboratory sleep

	On medication					Off medication				
	First night	First 3 nights	First 5 nights	Remaining nights	All nights	First night	First 3 nights	Second 3 nights	Remaining nights	Last night
Time awake	31.1	29.8	26.7	32.3	28.7	29.4	44.3	40.4	61.5	69.6
(30-sec pages)	(−22.6)	(−25.5)*	(−30.0)**	(−5.5)	(−20.5)*	(−28.3)	(+4.4)	(+6.2)	(+23.8)	(+33.8)
Number of awakenings	2.9	2.0	1.9	1.4	1.7	1.5	2.3	3.0	5.5	7.1
	(−0.6)	(−1.2)	(−1.2)	(−0.9)	(−1.1)	(−1.5)*	(−1.0)	(−0.7)	(+2.6)*	(+4.8)
Sleep latency	17.6	18.3	16.0	17.4	16.6	19.9	21.6	15.8	26.3	26.0
(30-sec pages)	(−9.1)	(−6.7)	(−7.5)	(−1.4)	(−4.8)	(+1.0)	(+2.1)	(−2.4)	(+1.5)	(+3.4)
Total sleep time	917	885	857	816	843	830	807	826	805	780
(30-sec pages)	(+56.8)**	(+40.6)	(+13.9)	(−16.7)	(+2.6)	(+13.3)	(−19.7)	(−20.8)	(−19.7)	(−46.8)
Stage 1	27.3	25.0	23.2	23.3	23.1	17.1	27.9	32.1	43.7	54.3
(30-sec pages)	(−8.3)	(−9.8)	(−13.5)	(−12.4)*	(−13.4)**	(−10.1)*	(−1.3)	(+1.4)	(+14.4)*	(+25.8)*
Stage 2	516	527	524	546	531	504	484	432	403	367
(30-sec pages)	(+101.4)***	(+97.8)***	(+97.6)***	(+127.6)***	(+107.2)***	(+64.0)	(+42.4)	(+19.6)	(−39.6)*	(−59.5)***
Stage 3	82.1	75.6	76.7	61.7	71.7	85.8	67.4	73.4	78.4	74.9
(30-sec pages)	(−15.4)	(−2.1)	(+0.2)	(−17.5)*	(−5.8)	(+20.8)	(−1.9)	(+6.3)	(+7.7)	(+0.0)
Stage 4	76.4	56.5	45.0	23.9	38.0	28.8	39.1	67.4	84.9	102
(30-sec pages)	(−9.0)	(−36.8)*	(−46.9)**	(−57.6)***	(−49.8)**	(−59.3)***	(−41.4)	(−32.4)***	(−8.0)	(+9.5)
Slow-wave sleep	159	132	122	856	110	115	106	141	163	176
(30-sec pages)	(−24.4)	(−38.8)	(−46.7)*	(−75.0)***	(−55.5)*	(−38.5)	(−43.3)*	(−26.1)	(−0.3)	(−0.3)
D-Time	215	200.7	189	161	178.9	184	188	221	194	182
(30-sec pages)	(−12.0)	(−8.6)	(−23.6)*	(−56.8)*	(−35.7)*	(−2.1)	(−17.5)	(−15.8)	(+5.9)	(−22.5)
D-Latency	227	230	226	238	231	242	226	162	162	144
(30-sec pages)	(+51.8)	(+46.0)	(+44.6)	(+57.7)*	(+51.8)*	(+72.3)*	(+55.6)*	(+20.6)*	(−18.9)	(−67.2)
Number of D-periods	4.8	4.3	4.1	3.5	3.9	3.9	3.7	4.0	4.3	4.8
	(+0.6)	(+0.3)	(+0.1)	(−0.7)*	(−0.2)	(−0.3)	(−0.4)*	(−0.3)	(+0.4)*	(+1.1)*
Number of stage shifts	52.8	45.6	45.1	35.3	42.0	41.8	45.3	49.5	62.2	70.4
	(−2.9)	(−9.9)**	(−10.6)**	(−21.9)**	(−14.5)***	(−12.4)*	(−8.7)	(−8.0)	(+5.5)	(+14.0)*
Cycle length	177	187	191	210	198	202	198	211	198	174
(30-sec pages)	(−30.9)**	(−17.6)***	(−13.8)***	(+14.5)	(−3.8)	(+2.4)	(−3.8)	(+7.7)	(−12.3)	(−51.3)*
Number of body movements	44.5	40.4	36.9	30.3	34.5	33.8	33.8	40.4	49.3	47.3
	(+2.6)	(−7.0)**	(−10.6)***	(−13.8)**	(−11.7)***	(−11.0)	(−10.4)***	(−4.3)	(+1.3)	(+0.4)
Disturbance index	75.6	70.2	63.6	62.5	63.2	63.1	78.2	80.8	111	117
	(−20.0)	(−32.6)**	(−40.6)***	(−19.4)	(−32.1)**	(−39.3)*	(−6.0)	(+1.9)	(+25.1)	(+34.3)

• $P < 0.05$; •• $P < 0.01$; ••• $P < 0.001$. Numbers in parentheses indicate drug mean minus placebo mean.
For notes on Table 1, see page 000: "Home log variables."

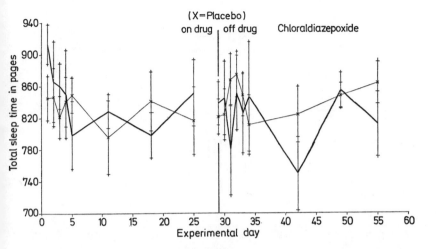

Fig. 1. Effects of chlordiazepoxide on total sleep time

drug administration and shows a decrease 1 to 2 weeks after discontinuation.

Effects on D-time are likewise definite and long-lasting: D-time is slightly but significantly reduced the first days and is further reduced for the following weeks. However, D-time returns to normal levels immediately on drug discontinuation, or possibly toward the end of the drug administration period (Fig. 3). There is no "rebound" increase. The curve for D-percent (Fig. 4) is fairly similar to that for total D-time. D-latency is significantly increased throughout the time of drug administration, with recovery occurring several days after discontinuation, again with no "rebound" (Fig. 5).

Number of body movements, number of stage shifts, and the "disturbance index" (a compound measure involving awakenings and body movements) are all very significantly decreased during administration of chlordiazepoxide and tend to remain decreased for some time after discontinuation.

Effects on Home Log Variables. Quality of sleep was judged significantly better on CDX than on placebo for the first two weeks on medication; there is no difference from placebo after

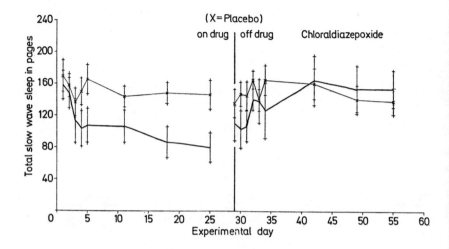

Fig. 2. Effects of chlordiazepoxide on slow-wave sleep

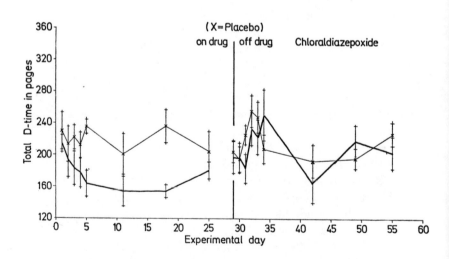

Fig. 3. Effects of chlordiazepoxide on D-time

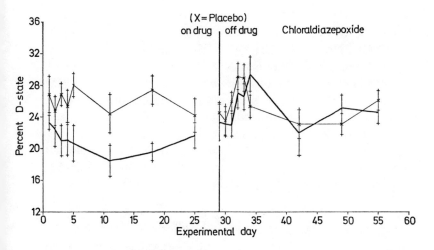

Fig. 4. Effects of chlordiazepoxide on percent D-time

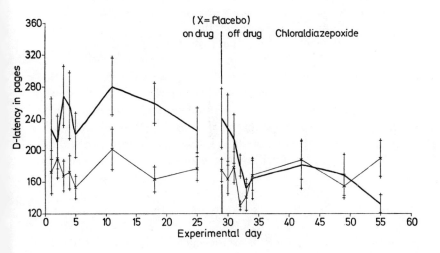

Fig. 5. Effects of chlordiazepoxide on D-latency

discontinuation. Subjects tended to feel slightly worse in the morning during CDX administration, with a significant worsening for two weeks after discontinuation. Administration of CDX produced no change in the number of "feel sick" responses, but discontinuation produced a significant increase. None of the POMS scales were significantly affected by CDX. Only one, the "fatigue" scale showed a trend toward greater fatigue both early on medication, late on medication, and after discontinuation (Table 2).

Effect on Interrelationship. On the whole, there were not many changes in interrelationships within laboratory variables, within home log variables, or between the two.

CONCLUSIONS AND DISCUSSION

This study shows that CDX, 50 mg per night, did have remarkably strong effects on the organization of sleep: slow-wave sleep—especially stage 4 sleep—and D-time were both significantly reduced throughout the time of drug administration (after the first days). The effects on slow-wave sleep were more marked than those found with any of the other medications studied. The reduction in D-time was greater than that of the other drugs, except for amitriptyline. What should be noted about CDX is that these effects increased rather than decreased with time; the body certainly did not appear to show tolerance to these effects of CDX as it did, for instance, with reserpine. This suggests that the reduction in D (and in SWS) is produced in a manner that does not allow homeostatic restoration within days or weeks—presumably in a manner not involving simple changes in catecholamines levels, for instance, since these are quickly restituted (Coulter, Lester, and Williams, 1971; see also our discussion of the effects of reserpine, Hartmann and Cravens, 1973 b). The reduction in SWS and especially stage 4 was long-lasting, with little evidence of tolerance. This suggests that SWS, although obtained in very constant amounts by normal subjects (Webb and Agnew, Jr., 1968; Webb, 1969)

Table 2. Chlordiazepoxide: Effects on home log variables

	On medication					Off medication				
	First week	Second week	Third week	Fourth week	All weeks	First week	Second week	Third week	Fourth week	All weeks
Estimated total sleep time (in hours and tenths)	7.3 (−0.3)	7.9 (+0.1)	7.5 (−0.1)	6.7 (+0.1)	7.6 (−0.1)	7.5 (+0.1)	7.3 (−0.3)	6.4 (−1.1)	6.4 (−0.3)	7.5 (−0.0)
Quality of sleep (1 = worst to 5 = best)	3.3 (+0.5)*	3.2 (+0.3)*	3.2 (+0.2)	2.6 (+0.0)	3.2 (+0.3)*	2.8	2.7	2.6	2.5	2.9
How feel in the morning (1 = worst to 5 = best)	2.7 (−0.2)	2.8 (−0.1)	2.8 (−0.2)**	2.5 (−0.1)	2.8 (−0.2)	2.7 (−0.1)	2.6 (−0.4)*	2.6 (−0.2)	2.5 (−0.1)	2.8 (−0.1)
Feel sick in any way (mean number of positive responses)	0.2 (−0.1)	0.3 (+0.1)	0.2 (+0.1)	0.1 (+0.1)	0.2 (+0.0)	0.3 (+0.2)*	0.3 (+0.3)*	0.1 (+0.0)	0.0 (+0.0)	0.2 (+0.2)*
Unusual psychological feelings (mean number of positive responses)	0.1 (−0.1)	0.1 (+0.1)	0.0 (−0.1)	0.0 (+0.0)	0.1 (−0.0)	0.1 (+0.1)	0.2 (+0.1)	0.0 (−0.1)	0.0 (−0.0)	0.1 (−0.0)
Fault of medication (mean number of positive responses—this refers to the two immediately preceding items and was only answered if there was a positive response to either)	0.3 (+0.2)	0.1 (+0.1)	0.0 (+0.0)	0.0 (+0.0)	0.2 (+0.0)	0.1 (+0.1)	0.0 (−0.0)	0.0 (+0.0)	0.0 (+0.0)	0.0 (+0.0)
Psychiatric Outpatient Mood Scale										
Tension-anxiety	−1.5 (−0.8)	−2.7 (−0.8)	−2.4 (−1.2)	0.6 (+1.5)	−1.6 (−0.3)	−0.1 (+1.0)	−0.7 (−0.2)	−1.9 (−0.4)	−1.8 (+0.5)	−1.4 (−0.6)
Anger-hostility	−8.9 (+0.0)	−0.9 (−0.4)	−9.8 (−0.5)	−7.9 (+0.1)	−9.4 (−0.3)	−8.6 (−1.3)	8.3 (−0.9)	−8.6 (−2.2)	−8.6 (−3.0)	−8.4 (−2.0)
Fatigue	0.0 (+4.2)	−2.3 (+1.6)	−1.2 (+3.3)	2.2 (+6.0)	−0.6 (+3.6)	−0.1 (+3.6)	−1.7 (+0.9)	−3.1 (+0.0)	−2.1 (+1.3)	−1.6 (0.6)
Depression	−9.3 (−0.8)	−11.2 (−3.1)	−11.3 (−3.0)	−4.3 (+3.0)	−10.1 (−1.8)	−7.1 (+0.0)	−9.7 (−3.2)	−9.5 (−0.9)	−9.0 (−0.1)	−9.4 (−2.7)
Vigor	5.6 (−2.8)	8.6 (+2.3)	6.8 (−0.4)	4.4 (+1.7)	6.7 (−0.1)	7.1 (+2.0)	7.6 (+1.1)	6.3 (−0.9)	5.4 (−2.9)	7.0 (0.6)
Confusion	1.8 (+1.3)	−0.1 (−0.7)	−0.3 (−1.3)	1.9 (+0.8)	0.8 (+0.0)	1.0 (−0.2)	0.2 (−1.0)	−0.9 (+0.3)	−0.1 (+1.5)	0.3 (−0.8)

* P < 0.05; ** P < 0.01; *** P < 0.001. Numbers in parentheses indicate drug mean minus placebo mean.
For notes on Table 2, see page 000: "Home log variables."

as well as by subjects with unusual total sleep time (Hartmann, Baekeland, Zwilling, and Hoy, 1971), is nonetheless amenable to long-term alteration without close negative-feedback control.

On the other hand, the effects of CDX on total sleep and waking lasted only one to three days, with rapid return to placebo levels, suggesting that these parameters are maintained under closer feedback control. The early *increase* of total sleep while D and SWS are *decreasing*, as well as the differing time-course, strongly suggest that the effect of CDX on total sleep versus waking involves different brain mechanisms than the effect on D and SWS discussed above.

We have assumed above that the decreases in slow-wave sleep and D-time are primary effects, and thus that increase in stage 2 was secondary (i.e., stage 2 merely filled up space). However, the dramatic increases in stage 2, reaching higher significance levels than the other changes, suggest at least the possibility that CDX may have a primary effect in increasing stage 2 time.

If D-time and/or slow-wave sleep are produced in response to some need, as is suggested by the phenomenon of rebound increase after deprivation, then it could be possible to decrease the need pharmacologically. Perhaps the tranquilization produced by CDX is the primary effect, and the reduction of D-time and slow-wave sleep may be a secondary effect resulting from a reduced need for D and slow-wave sleep. The fact that CDX, to our surprise, produced prolonged reduction in D-time and slow-wave sleep without any rebound increase in either one, might be seen as lending support to the notion that it somehow reduced the body's requirement for these portions of sleep.

However, considering the very dramatic effects on laboratory sleep, combined with relatively little effect on the home log variables and mood variables,[1] it seems improbable that

1. Of the five drugs studied in this long-term design, CDX can be characterized as producing the greatest alteration in the laboratory sleep variables, but with almost no alteration in home log variables.

the primary effect should be on psychological state or mood, followed by a sleep effect.[2] Rather, I believe we have demonstrated one or several direct and long-lasting central nervous system effects.

It seems possible that CDX exerts its effect on sleep by some specific neurophysiological mechanism, somehow reducing the activity of centers or systems that produce SWS as well as systems that produce D. The suggestion that CDX interferes with electrical activity in the brainstem (Przybyla and Wang, 1968; Goodman and Gilman, 1970) is in a general sense compatible with our findings: an overall reduction of discharge or activity in the ARAS, as found on short-term administration, would be likely to produce decreased waking and increased total sleep, as indeed was found in the first days of drug administration.

If the findings of Wise et al. (1972) with the benzodiazepine oxazepam are also true of CDX, we might explain our long-term findings along the following lines: early during drug administration, ARAS activity is diminished, along with a diminished turnover of catecholamines as well as serotonin. Since ARAS activity, including activity of norepinephrine and dopamine, is strongly implicated in maintaining wakefulness (Jones, Bobillier, and Jouvet, 1969; Hartmann, 1970), the early effect of CDX is a shift toward more sleep and less waking. The catecholamine changes are usually compensated for in a few days (catecholamine turnover returns to normal); however, serotonin turnover remains low for a longer time (Wise et al., 1972) and this could be related to the decrease in SWS and D-time. Serotonin is probably involved in maintaining normal sleep as a whole. There may be species differences here; in the cat, serotonin has been suggested to be related especially to S-sleep; in man, agents which increase serotonin

2. We also investigated whether the effects could be indirect in another sense—perhaps CDX changed the amount the subject exercised or smoked, or the extent to which he became ill, etc., and these secondarily produced changes in sleep. Our data on these points revealed nothing that could explain the present findings.

activity have been shown to increase D-time in several studies (Oswald, 1964; Hartmann, Chung, and Chien, 1971; Griffiths, Lester, Coulter, and Williams, 1972), increase SWS in others (Griffiths et al., 1972; Hartmann and Cravens, to be published), and also appears to maintain the structure and regular cyclic activity of sleep as a whole (Cohen, Ferguson, Henriksen, Stolk, Zarcone, Barchas, and Dement, 1970; Hartmann, 1973). Thus the reduced SWS and D-time found might be compatible with a reduced serotonin turnover; but this is very tentative at present.

Certainly long-term sleep studies represent one clear-cut and sensitive measure of CNS changes, and on this basis it is certain that long-term CDX in a clinical dosage range produced some profound CNS changes. This study demonstrates that CDX is not a placebo, and in fact in terms of changes in sleep EEG, it must be considered a very potent drug.

The clinical question of the use of benzodiazepines as hypnotics can, of course, not be settled by a study of this kind, since the subjects were not insomniacs, and only a single dosage level of one benzodiazepine was investigated.

It must be kept in mind that there is little or no evidence demonstrating that altering sleep EEG patterns produces any clear-cut detrimental effects or subjective feelings of poor sleep. It is somewhat ironic that over the last ten years, as EEG sleep studies have become more prominent, barbiturates and some of the older hypnotics have been looked upon with disfavor because of their disruptive effect on EEG sleep patterns, while one of the benzodiazepines, flurazepam, is becoming increasingly popular, in part because of promotion indicating that this drug will not produce these alterations in sleep patterns. From the present study it is clear that CDX produces very profound changes in EEG sleep patterns on long-term administration. It appears from other studies that flurazepam and other benzodiazepines probably produce similar alterations. Nonetheless, sleep was subjectively rated as quite good with CDX in this study.

This work was supported in part by National Institute of Mental Health Grant # MH 14520.

References

Cohen, H. B., Ferguson, J. M., Henriksen, S. J., Stolk, J. M., Zarcone, V. J., Barchas, J. D., Dement, W. C.: Effects of chronic depletion of brain serotonin on sleep and behavior. Proc. Amer. Psychol. Ass. 78, 831–832 (1970)

Coulter, J. D., Lester, B. J., Williams, H. L.: Reserpine and sleep. Psychopharmacologia (Berl.) 19, 134–147 (1971)

Ehrhart, C.: (Action of oxazepam 50 on sleep disorders) Action de l'oxatepam 50 sur les troubles du sommeil. Lyon Méd. 225, 1173–1175 (1971) (Fre.)

Fisher, C., Byrne, J., Edwards, A., Kahn, E.: A psychophysiological study of nightmares. J. Amer. Psychoanal. Ass. 18, 747–782 (1970)

Glick, B. S., Schulman, D., Turecki, S.: Diazepam (VALIUM) treatment in childhood sleep disorders: A preliminary investigation. Dis. Nerv. Syst. 32, 565–566 (1971)

Goodman, L. S., Gilman, A. (Eds.): The pharmacological basis of therapeutics. Fourth Edition. London-Toronto: Macmillan Comp. 1970

Griffiths, W. J., Lester, B. K., Coulter, J. D., Williams, H. L.: Tryptophan and sleep in young adults. Psychophysiology 9, 345–356 (1972)

Haider, I., Oswald, I.: Effects of amylobarbitone and nitrazepam on the electrodermogram and other features of sleep. Brit. J. Psychiat. 118, 519–522 (1971)

Hartmann, E.: The effect of four drugs on sleep in man. Psychopharmacologia (Berl.) 12, 346–353 (1968)

Hartmann, E.: The D-state and norepinephrine-dependent systems. In: Sleep and Dreaming, E. Hartmann (Ed.), pp. 308–328. Boston: Little, Brown & Co. 1970

Hartmann, E.: Effects of l-tryptophane on sleep: Human and animal studies. In: (Proceedings of the Würzburg Symposium, The nature of sleep, September 1971) The Nature of Sleep, pp. 290–295. Basel: S. Karger 1973

Hartmann, E., Baekeland, F., Zwilling, G., Hoy, P.: Sleep need: How much sleep and what kind? Amer. J. Psychiat. **127**, 1001–1008 (1971)

Hartmann, E., Chung, R., Chien, C.: L-tryptophane and sleep. Psychopharmacologia (Berl.) **19**, 114–127 (1971)

Hartmann, E., Cravens, J.: The effects of long-term administration of psychotropic drugs on human sleep: I. Methodology and the effects of placebo. Psychopharmacologia (Berl.) **33**, 153–167 (1973 a)

Hartmann, E., Cravens, J.: The effects of long-term administration of psychotropic drugs on human sleep: II. The effects of reserpine. Psychopharmacologia (Berl.) **33**, 169–184 (1973 b)

Hartmann, E., Cravens, J.: Hypnotic effects of l-tryptophane. (To be published)

Jones, B. E., Bobillier, P., Jouvet, M.: Effets de la destruction des neurones contenant des catecholamines du mesencephale sur le cycle veillesommeils du chat. C. R. Soc. Biol. (Paris) **163**, 176–180 (1969)

Kales, A., Allen, C., Scharf, M. B., Kales, J. D.: Hypnotic drugs and their effectiveness. All-night EEG studies of insomniac subjects. Arch. Gen. Psychiat. **23**, 226–232 (1970)

Kales, A., Kales, J. D., Scharf, M. B., Tan, T.-L.: Hypnotics and altered sleep-dream patterns. 2. All-night EEG studies of chloral hydrate, flurazepam, and methaqualone. Arch. Gen. Psychiat. **23**, 219–225 (1970)

Kales, J., Kales, A., Bixler, E. O., Slyde, E. S.: Effects of placebo and flurazepam on sleep patterns in insomniac subjects. Clin. Pharmacol. Ther. **12**, 691–697 (1971)

Monti, J. M., Trenchi, H. M., Morales, F.: (Effects of a benzodiazepine derivative, RO 5-4200, on the EEG and the sleep cycle in insomniacs) Acciones de un derivado benzodiazepinico, el RO 5-4200 sobre el EEG y el ciclo de sueno en pacientes con insomnio. Acta neurol. lat.-amer. **17**, 5–11 (1971)

Oswald, I.: Effect of l-tryptophane upon human sleep. Electroenceph. Clin. Neurophysiol. **17**, 603–604 (1964)

Przybyla, A. C., Wang, S. C.: Locus of central depressant action of diazepam. J. Pharmacol. Exp. Ther. **163**, 439–447 (1968)

Randall, L. O.: Pharmacology of chlordiazepoxide (LIBRIUM). Dis. Nerv. Syst. **22**, 7–15 (1961)

Rickels, K.: Drug use in outpatient treatment. Amer. J. Psychiat. **124**, 20–31 (1968)

Webb, W. B.: The nature of all night sleep patterns. Activ. nerv. sup. (Praha) **11**, 90–97 (1969)

Webb, W. B., Agnew, H. W., Jr.: Measurement and characteristics of nocturnal sleep. Progr. Clin. Psychol. **8**, 2–27 (1968)

Wise, C. C., Berger, B. D., Stein, L.: Benzodiazepines: Anxiety-reducing activity by reduction of serotonin turnover in the brain. Science **177**, 180–183 (1972)

Appendix B

The Effects of Drugs on Sleep: A Clinical Study of Sleeping Medication

Here we reproduce one of a number of clinical studies investigating the effects of hypnotic medication. I believe that although sleep laboratory studies can give us some important detailed information about effects on sleep, evaluation of hypnotic medication clearly also requires its evaluation in a group of insomniacs who would normally be taking such medication. Usually such studies must involve a large number of patients in order to detect systematic differences between drugs and placebo despite great differences among individual patients, large placebo effects, and so on. Thus, because of the expense and inconvenience of all-night sleep recordings, these clinical investigations usually cannot be laboratory studies.

In the present study, triazolam, secobarbitol, and placebo are compared in a population of insomniac patients. Triazolam is a benzodiazepine, related to flurazepam and diazepam. Secobarbital (Seconal) is the most widely used barbiturate hypnotic. The results of this study are important in themselves, and in addition this investigation demonstrates interesting aspects of drug research design. Such clinical studies are a significant part of the overall evaluation of hypnotic medication. The sleep laboratory is not used; thus, the dependent variables (outcome measures) are basically the patient's subjective report of how well he slept and felt, rated in several ways by the patient and by his physician.

Triazolam in Insomniac Family Practice Patients*

Karl Rickels, M.D., Russell L. Gingrich, Jr., M.D., Richard
J. Morris, M.D., Howard Rosenfeld, M.D., Milton M.
Perloff, M.D., E. L. Clark, M.D., and Ann Schilling, A.B.

*The Departments of Psychiatry, University of Pennsylvania,
and Philadelphia General Hospital*

Abstract. Triazolam, 0.5 mg, a benzodiazepine with hypnotic
properties, was compared to secobarbital, 100 mg, and placebo in a 1-week study conducted with 100 insomniac family
practice patients. Considerable sensitivity to differential treatment effects was demonstrated for these family practice patients as well as for a research methodology that combines a
crossover design, permitting preference ratings, with a between-patient design. In almost all sleep parameters, assessed
with a variety of subjective techniques, triazolam and secobarbital were shown to be significantly more effective than
placebo. Triazolam was consistently and often significantly
indicated to be a more effective hypnotic, particularly for reducing nocturnal awakening, than secobarbital. Analysis of
self-report emotional distress data revealed that present insomniac patients were slightly more emotionally symptomatic
than other nonpsychiatric populations. Triazolam was followed
by the greatest and secobarbital by the least relief of emotional symptoms, and triazolam emerged as an especially effective hypnotic for initially more depressed insomniac patients. Present findings suggest that type and degree of
emotional symptomatology may affect the response of insomniac patients to hypnotics.

Triazolam, a substituted benzodiazepine, has been shown to
have hypnotic activity in man. In Veterans Administration
Hospital inpatients, Wang and Stockdale[15] found 1.0 mg of

* Reprinted with permission from *Clin. Pharmacol. Ther.* 18 (1975):
315–24. Copyrighted by The C. V. Mosby Company, St. Louis, Missouri,
U.S.A.

triazolam to be equal or superior to either 15 or 30 mg of flurazepam in duration and depth of sleep and in reduction of nocturnal awakenings. In a sleep laboratory experiment, using a crossover design, Roth, Kramer, and Schwartz[12] found sleep induction to be more rapid with triazolam than with placebo. Matta and associates[8] reported that triazolam, 0.5 mg, was a more effective sleep inducer than flurazepam, 30 mg, and was superior to placebo in induction, duration of sleep, reduction of nocturnal awakenings, and quality of sleep in presurgical patients.

The present 7-day, double-blind study was designed in 2 parts: Part A using triazolam 0.5 mg and placebo; Part B using secobarbital sodium, 100 mg, and placebo. The purposes

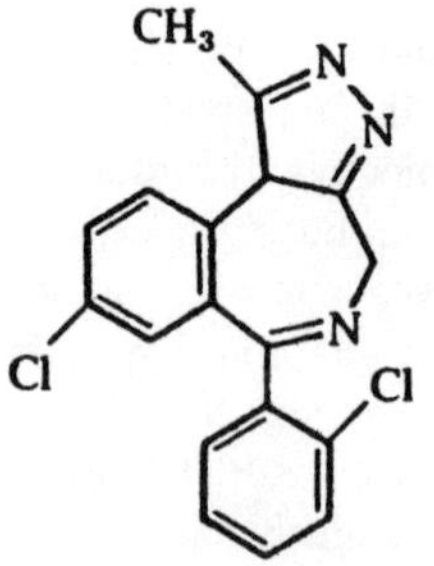

Fig. 1. Structural formula for triazolam.

of this study were (1) to evaluate the safety and efficacy of triazolam (0.5 mg) in insomniac family practice patients, (2) to compare its results to those obtained with secobarbital (100 mg) in the same treatment setting, (3) to assess the sensitivity with which insomniac private family practice outpatients, i.e., those patients who are the primary consumers of hypnotics, detect the differences between hypnotic agents and placebo, and (4) to search for a possible relationship between emotional distress level and treatment response.

METHOD

Subjects The study sample consisted of 100 outpatients attending the offices of 14 family practitioners. Patients had a history of insomnia and current difficulties in falling sleep or remaining asleep throughout the night. Fifty patients each participated in parts A and B of the study. Patients were able to communicate intelligently with the physician, and informed consent was obtained. Excluded from the study were patients with organic diseases not well controlled, patients with emotional illness requiring psychotropic medication, patients with a history of drug abuse or excessive use of sedatives, and pregnant or lactating females.

Demographic characteristics were similar for all 4 treatment groups (i.e., triazolam and placebo, secobarbital and placebo). Patients were predominantly white (84%), married (64%), and female (78%), with at least a high school education (58%). The mean age was 48 years. Coffee usage was moderate, with 57% drinking 3 or more cups a day. Half of the patients smoked cigarettes, with most using a pack or less a day.

Variables relating to current patterns of sleep disturbance as well as illness history are given in Table I. A variety of sleep problems were reported by these family practice patients. They not only had difficulty falling asleep, but also suffered from nocturnal as well as early awakenings, and 76% stated that they began their day feeling tired. It is interesting to note that when patients were asked to specify a precipitating event they could link with the onset of their insomnia, 15% cited social stress, 13% physical illness, and 30% miscellaneous reasons, while 42% were unable to define any precipitating cause. Approximately half of the patients had taken medication previously for their insomnia. Of those, 14 had used barbiturates, 5 had taken antihistamines, such as diphenhydramine or over-the-counter (OTC) sleep aids; 2 had taken flurazepam; and 29 had used various other medications, including chloral hydrate. Most (84%) patients expected hyp-

Table 1

Sleep disturbance in insomniac family practice patients (N = 100)

Current pattern	N	Illness history	N
Difficulties falling asleep		*Onset of present sleep*	
≤30 min	26	*problems*	
31–60 min	27	≤3 mo	29
>60 min	47	>3–12 mo	23
		>12 mo	48
Awakenings during night			
None	9	*Course of sleep problems*	
1–2	31	Constant	66
≥3	60	Cyclic, intermittent	32
Awakening early		*Number of previous hypnotics*	
Yes	87	*in past 3 Yr*	
No	13	None	46
		One	27
Usual length of sleep		<2	25
≤4 hr	26		
>4–6 hr	47	*Last hypnotic helped:*	
>6–7 hr	18	A lot, quite a bit	27
>7 hr	9	A little, not at all	26
Feeling sleepy in A.M.			
Yes	76		
No	24		
Predominant type of insomnia			
Difficulty falling asleep	45		
Awakening during night	42		
Awakening early	13		

notic drug therapy, 78% had a positive attitude toward medication, and 59% received a good prognosis from their physicians.

Medication   Medication in Part A was prepared in tablet form containing either 0.5 mg triazolam or placebo identical in appearance. Medication in Part B was prepared in capsule form containing either 100 mg of secobarbital or placebo identical in appearance. All patients received a package of small bottles, each containing one tablet or one capsule. Bottles were clearly marked by day. Patients were instructed to use the bottles consecutively and to take their medication at bedtime.

Design and analysis   The study design was double-blind, with systematized random allocation of medication within Part A and Part B (Table II). Patients were assigned serially within Part A and Part B. The first 2 days of the study made use of a crossover design that allowed for a preference test as described by Jick[5] and by Zimmerman.[16] The patient then continued taking the medication received on day 2 for the remaining 5 days of the study. Days 2 to 7 can therefore be considered a between-patient design.

Data were analyzed only for those patients who completed more than one day of treatment. In Part A, 24 patients were treated with triazolam and 26 with placebo. In Part B, 26 patients were treated with secobarbital and 24 with placebo. Treatment group pertains to the medication received in the between-patient part of the study from days 2 to 7. Since data analyses showed no significant pretreatment or treatment response differences between the 2 placebo groups, all statistical analyses reported in the paper, with the exception of those conducted for preference ratings, were carried out with both placebo groups combined. It should also be noted that only

Table 2

Study design

	Part A (T = triazolam, 0.5 mg.; P = placebo)						
	Day						
	1	2	3	4	5	6	7
N = 24	P	T	T	T	T	T	T
N = 26	T	P	P	P	P	P	P
	Part B (S = secobarbital, 100 mg.; P = placebo)						
N = 26	P	S	S	S	S	S	S
N = 24	S	P	P	P	P	P	P

data for patients who stated they actually took their medication were included in these analyses.

Clinical measures.   The first was the *Intake Information Form,* on which various demographic and attitudinal variables, sleep history, intercurrent medical or psychiatric illness, and treatment data were recorded by the physician at the first study visit.

The *Daily Sleep Questionnaire Booklet (SQB)* was completed by the patient daily following breakfast, and contained the items shown in Table III. On the second day, an additional page contained the following preference question: "Which night did you have the better night's sleep? Night 1, Night 2, No preference." Patients were instructed to return the booklet at their next visit, usually one week after onset of the study. The first question for each day, allowing the patient to be truthful about whether or not he or she took the medication, may be seen as contributing to the reliability of the present data.

On the *Physician Sleep Questionnaire (PSQ),* the physician, at the end of the study, recorded the patient's overall evaluation of medication efficacy during days 2 to 7 in such target areas as sleep latency, quality of dreams, number of hours slept, side reactions, and number of nocturnal awakenings.

The *Hopkins Symptom Checklist (HSCL)*[1] was completed by the patient at both visits and contained 35 items rated on a scale of (1) "not at all" to (4) "extremely." The scale provided 5 major factors, i.e., Somatization, Obsession-Compulsion (Performance Difficulty), Interpersonal Sensitivity, Depression, and Anxiety, and a total score.

The *Clyde Mood Scale (CMS)* was a 48-item self-report checklist designed by Clyde[3] and yielded 6 factors.

Laboratory tests (i.e., hematology, blood chemistry, and urinalysis) were performed before and after treatment whenever possible. Responses within the normal range were found in all instances.

Table 3

Sleep questionnaire booklet (SQB) items

Did you take medication?	How did you sleep last night?

Did you take medication?
1. Yes
2. No

How much did medicine help you sleep last night?
1. A lot
2. Quite a bit
3. A little
4. Did not sleep

Sleep onset (latency)
1. <15 min
2. <30 min
3. <1 hr
4. >1 hr

Take nap yesterday?
1. Yes
2. No

Number of awakenings during night (incidences)

Number of hr sleep (in hr)

Compared to usual sleep:
1. Longer than usual
2. As long as usual
3. Shorter than usual

How did you sleep last night?
(Depth)
1. Deeply
2. Medium
3. Lightly

Quality of sleep:
1. Very good
2. Good
3. Fair
4. Poor
5. Terrible

How did you feel when you awoke this morning?
1. More rested
2. Same as usual
3. Less rested

Did you dream?
1. Yes
2. No

Were dreams
1. Pleasant
2. Unpleasant
3. Do not know

Side effects from medicine?
1. Yes
2. No

RESULTS AND DISCUSSION

Completion rate A completer was defined as a patient who completed the Sleep Questionnaire Booklet (SQB) on all 7 days. Using this stringent criterion, 22 (92%) of triazolam, 23 (88%) of secobarbital, and 38 (76%) of placebo patients were designated as completers. The differences in completion rate were not statistically significant, although a trend was noted at the 20% level in favor of active drugs over placebo.

Side effects   Side effects attributed by the patient to medication were recorded daily on the SQB. By far the most frequently reported side effects were drowsiness, dizziness or weakness, grogginess, and fatigue. For presentation purposes, these symptoms have been combined to form a sedation cluster and are presented by day in Table IV. Since "grogginess" and "headaches" were suggested as side effects on the SQB, the incidence of these reported side

Table 4

Number of patients reporting side effects by day
(figures given in percent)

		Day 2			Day 3			Day 4		
		T	S	P	T	S	P	T	S	P
Side effect	*N =*	24	26	47	24	25	48	24	25	45
Sedation (drowsiness, dizziness, weakness, grogginess, fatigue)		46	8	19*	21	16	12	29	20	7†
Grogginess‡			8	15		12	2		8	7
Headaches‡		12	19	11	4	8	6	12	20	11

		Day 5			Day 6			Day 7		
		T	S	P	T	S	P	T	S	P
Side effect	*N =*	21	24	40	22	23	37	21	23	38
Sedation (drowsiness, dizziness, weakness, grogginess, fatigue)		24	17	2†	23	13	5	24	4	5†
Grogginess‡		14	8	2	23	9	3	14	0	5
Headaches‡		5	12	8	0	13	8	5	4	5

* $p < 0.01$.
† $p < 0.05$.
‡ Suggested to the patient as possible side effects on SQB.

effects is probably inflated and data for these 2 specific side effects are therefore also shown in Table IV. "Grogginess" is seen to contribute heavily to the sedation cluster. The reporting of sedation and grogginess is particularly marked for triazolam, and slightly less for secobarbital than for placebo, at day 2. While sedation and grogginess decrease for triazolam patients following day 2, these side effects are reported more frequently by triazolam than by either secobarbital or placebo patients at all study days. With secobarbital, there is some increase in sedation following day 2, a decrease in sedation by day 7, and a slight tendency for headaches to be reported more frequently than with either triazolam or placebo.

Preference ratings of hypnotic efficacy. By day 2 each patient had received either triazolam and placebo or secobarbital and placebo. Preference data, given in Table V, clearly indicate the superiority of both active drugs to placebo. When comparing preference ratings of Part A (triazolam-placebo) with Part B (secobarbital-placebo), one finds triazolam to be superior to secobarbital at the 10% level (triazolam-preference 80% and secobarbital preference 60%) ($\chi^2 = 3.62$, df 1).

Between-patient analyses of hypnotic efficacy. Treatment results for triazolam, secobarbital, and placebo (both placebo groups combined) were initially compared by applying a univariate analysis of variance technique to the mean SQB

Table 5

Preference rating after 2 days on study

	Part A	Part B
	Triazolam vs placebo (N = 49)	Secobarbital vs placebo (N = 50)
Patient preferred:		
Drug night	39	30
Placebo night	4	9
No preference	6	11
	z = 5.1849*	z = 3.2025*
	p = 0.00003	p < 0.00007

* Normal approximation of the binomial distribution.

responses for days 2 through 7. These results are presented in Table VI. It should be noted that data on dreaming are omitted since none of the medications had any consistent effect on this parameter. For all other SQB criteria assessed, Table VI shows a clear order of efficacy ranging from triazolam to secobarbital to placebo. With the Newman-Keuls statistic, it was found that both active agents were significantly more effective than placebo, and that triazolam was also more effective than secobarbital in the following variables: "How much did the medication help you sleep?" ($p < 0.10$), number of nocturnal awakenings ($p < 0.01$), and quality of sleep ($p < 0.05$).

Table 6

Sleep questionnaire booklet means: Days 2-7 combined

Variables[a]	Triazolam (N = 24)	Secobarbital (N = 24)	Placebo (N = 49)	(df 2, 95) Variate F ratio
How much did medicine help you sleep last night? (1-4)	1.87	2.29	2.94	17.20†
How long did it take you to fall asleep? (1-4)	2.00	2.41	2.83	6.99‡
How often did you wake up? (0-9)	0.42	1.70	2.22	18.67†
How many hours did you sleep? (hr)	6.75	6.25	5.00	12.46†
How was your sleep compared to usual sleep? (1-3)	1.50	1.69	2.07	13.02†
How deeply did you sleep? (1-3)	1.56	1.80	2.25	13.57†
How well did you sleep? (1-5)	1.87	2.33	3.04	21.39†
How did you feel in A.M. (1-3)	1.60	1.78	2.07	10.24†

[a] In all variables lower score indicates more improvement with the exception of "How many hours did you sleep?"
† $p < 0.001$.
‡ $p < 0.005$.

SQB data showing triazolam to be especially effective relative to secobarbital in reducing nocturnal awakenings, but not markedly different from secobarbital in terms of sleep induction, appear consistent with results reported for comparable agents by Andersen and Lingjaerde.[1] Several years ago, these authors found that the benzodiazepine nitrazepam exerted greater hypnotic effect than the barbiturate phenobarbital sodium in patients suffering from "frequent awakening," while phenobarbital was more effective in patients complaining primarily of "early insomnia."

The major parameters of the SQB were also used in a repeated measurement analysis of drug response for days 2 through 7. The pattern of response obtained in the 3 medication groups is graphically illustrated in Fig. 2 for "how much did the medication help you sleep last night?" and "sleep latency." In all variables, treatment differences were most marked at day 2 and decreased as the week progressed. This observation was supported by analyses of variance conducted for each day separately. The active drugs consistently produced more improvement than placebo, and the response to secobarbital was more variable and less favorable than the response to triazolam.

Selected variables from the Physician Sleep Questionnaire, completed at treatment end point, are presented in Table VII. As with the SQB, no medication differences were observed in either incidence or type of dreaming (47 patients reported dreaming during the one-week study period). Again, the order of efficacy ranges from triazolam to secobarbital to placebo. Significant (p < 0.10) differences between the 2 active agents emerged in measures assessing nocturnal awakening, sleep quality, and restful feeling in A.M.

Emotional distress   Information on emotional distress, as assessed with the patient-completed HSCL, is given in Table VIII. Pretreatment means are shown for the total sample because the individual treatment groups did not differ significantly in their initial HSCL scores. The emotional dis-

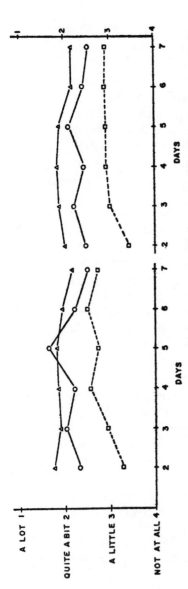

Fig. 2. Patterns of drug response: Repeated measurement analysis. Δ, Triazolam (N = 19); o, secobarbital (N = 20); □, placebo (N = 32). *Left*, How much did medication help you last night? (p < 0.012 linear). *Right*, Sleep latency (p < 0.020 linear).

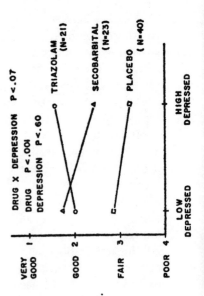

Fig. 3. Quality of sleep as a function of initial level of depression.

Table 7

Physician sleep assessment at treatment end point (figures in percent)

Variables	Triazolam (0.5 mg) (N = 21)	Secobarbital (100 mg) (N = 26)	Placebo (N = 50)	p < *
Duration:				
≦6 hr	10	23	51	0.01
>6 hr	90	77	49	
Awake during night (incidences):				
0-1	81	54	33	0.01
2-6	19	46	67	
Quality:				
Light	10	19	38	0.001
Medium	33	58	48	
Deep	57	23	14	
Restful feeling in A.M.:				
Less rested, Same as usual	24	54	65	0.01
More rested than usual	76	46	35	

* Based on chi square.

tress of these insomniac patients is lower than that of anxious outpatients (e.g., Depression factor, 2.04; Anxiety factor, 2.22),[4] but higher than that of "normal" gynecologic patients (e.g., Depression factor, 1.40; Anxiety factor, 1.32)[10] or obese family practice patients (e.g., Depression factor, 1.42; Anxiety factor, 1.34.)[11]

Change in emotional distress, as reflected in one week adjusted means derived from an analysis of covariance, is shown in Table VIII for the 3 medication groups. Triazolam is seen to be associated with the greatest, and secobarbital with the least, reduction in emotional distress. This tendency reaches significance in the HSCL Interpersonal Sensitivity and Depression factors. Some support for these results may be found in the observation by Schwartz, Kramer, and Roth[13] that triazolam did not significantly worsen mood in normal subjects, an effect that has been reported for the barbiturates.[6] Indeed, the present analysis indicated that triazolam was

Table 8

Emotional distress as affected by triazolam, secobarbital, and placebo

Checklist (HSCL) Hopkins Symptom factors	Pre-study means	One-week adjusted means			F ratio (df 2, 84)
		Triazolam (N = 22)	Secobarbital (N = 23)	Placebo (N = 43)	
1. Somatization	1.69	1.55	1.63	1.51	0.96
2. Obsession-compulsion	1.67	1.51	1.58	1.46	0.69
3. Interpersonal sensitivity	1.84	1.47	1.82	1.60	4.29°
4. Depression	1.88	1.50	1.78	1.63	4.21°
5. Anxiety	1.63	1.48	1.55	1.51	0.20
Total score	1.78	1.50	1.68	1.57	2.23

° $p < 0.025$.

particularly effective in alleviating emotional distress in patients who were initially more symptomatic, while secobarbital was not. This tendency was reflected in heterogeneity of regression effects, which reached significance in the Somatization ($p < 0.005$), Interpersonal Sensitivity ($p < 0.025$), and Depression ($p < 0.005$) factors, and in the total score ($p < 0.01$).

These HSCL data suggest that initial emotional distress, and particularly depression, may be related to treatment response. Evidence of such a relationship was found in an analysis conducted for patients divided above and below the median of the HSCL Depression factor when using "quality of sleep" as the outcome criterion. As shown in Fig. 3, a strong trend ($p < 0.07$, one-tailed) emerged for triazolam to exert greatest hypnotic effect in high-depressed, and for secobarbital to be most effective in low-depressed insomniac patients.

A final observation on the psychotropic effect of triazolam, derived from analyses of Clyde Mood Scale (CMS) data, is offered here because it replicates results obtained with another benzodiazepine several years ago.[9] Specifically, just as was found for chlordiazepoxide 40 mg/day and 80 mg/day, triazolam effected a significant increase in both the CMS Aggressive and Friendly factors, suggesting a benzodiazepine-induced increase in "assertiveness."

COMMENT

Present results clearly indicate, just as Beecher[2] and Lasagna[7] reported many years ago, that subjective responses can indeed be quantified when appropriate methodology, e.g., the double-blind, placebo control, randomization of treatment, and statistical data handling, is used. The data also show considerable sensitivity for a research design that incorporates the use of a crossover design, allowing for preference ratings, with a between-patient design. Furthermore, the study demonstrates that reliable and relevant data on hypnotic agents can be obtained within the family practice setting. This represents a most important finding, as the vast majority of hypnotic agents are prescribed for family practice patients, and as treatment agents should, whenever possible, be evaluated within the setting in which they are most commonly employed.

Indeed, marked sensitivity to differential treatment effects was found for the present insomniac family practice patients. They consistently reported greater efficacy for both triazolam, 0.5 mg, and secobarbital, 100 mg, than for placebo. Significant drug-placebo differences emerged in almost all sleep parameters, on daily patient measures as well as physician end point ratings, and in analyses assessing preference test data, mean treatment response data, and response pattern data (i.e., repeated measurement analyses). Present patients also discriminated among the 3 study medications in the reporting of side reactions, indicating sedation and grogginess to be most marked with triazolam.

The fact that these insomniac patients consistently, and sometimes significantly, indicated triazolam, 0.5 mg, to be a more effective hypnotic than secobarbital, 100 mg, may be seen as consistent with previous research. Thus Lasagna[7] as well as Urbach[14] have reported that secobarbital, 100 mg, assumes an intermediate position in efficacy between secobarbital, 200 mg, and placebo. Equating triazolam with secobarbital, 200 mg, a very similar pattern of response emerged in the present study.

Interestingly, present insomniac family practice patients appeared somewhat higher in emotional distress than such other nonpsychiatric samples as gynecologic[10] and obese[11] patients. Triazolam effected the greatest and secobarbital the least decrease in emotional symptoms, and triazolam represented an especially effective hypnotic, relative to secobarbital, in initially more depressed insomniac patients. Present data suggest that type and degree of emotional symptomatology may well emerge as important factors influencing the response of insomniac patients to hypnotic agents.

The authors thank Drs. Bernard Zamostien, Harry Dion, William Rial, Lester Sablosky, Edward Kelly, and Benjamin Schneider for participating in the data collection phase of the study; Mr. Norman Norstad for coordinating the study; and Ms. Janice Vlahovich for conducting the data analyses.

References

1. Andersen, T., and Lingjaerde, O.: Nitrazepam (Mogadan) as a sleep-inducing agent, Br. J. Psychiatr. 115: 1393–1397, 1969.
2. Beecher, H. K.: Measurement of subjective responses: Quantitative effects of drugs, London, 1959, Oxford University Press.
3. Clyde, D. J.: Manual for the Clyde Mood Scale, Coral Gables Fla., 1963, Biometric Laboratory, University of Miami.
4. Derogatis, L. R., Lipman, R. S., Rickels, K., Uhlenhuth, E. H., and Covi, L.: The Hopkins Symptom Checklist (HSCL): A measure of primary symptom dimensions, *in* Pichot, P., editor: Psychological measurements in psychopharmacology, Mod. Probl. Pharmacopsychiatry 7: 79–110, Basel, 1974, Karger.
5. Jick, H.: Clinical evaluation of hypnotics, *in* Kales, A., editor: Sleep: Physiology and pathology. A symposium, Philadelphia, 1969, J. B. Lippincott Co., pp. 289–297.

6. Kales, A., Malmstrom, E., and Tan, T.: Drugs and dreaming, *in* Abt, G., and Riess, D., editors: Progress in clinical psychology, New York, 1969, Grune & Stratton, Inc., vol. 8, pp. 154–167.
7. Lasagna, L.: A study of hypnotic drugs in patients with chronic diseases: Comparative efficacy of placebo; methaprylon (Noludar); meprobamate (Miltown, Equanil); pentobarbital; phenobarbital; secobarbital, J. Chron. Dis. 3: 122–133, 1956.
8. Matta, B., Franco, A. E., le Zotte, L. A., Rudzik, A. D., and Veldkamp, W.: Comparison of triazolam, flurazepam and placebo as hypnotic agents in pre-surgical patients. Curr. Ther. Res. 16: 958–963, 1974.
9. Rickels, K., and Clyde, D. J.: Clyde mood scale changes in anxious outpatients produced by chlordiazepoxide therapy, J. Nerv. Ment. Dis. 145: 154–157, 1967.
10. Rickels, K., Garcia, C.-R., and Fisher, E.: A measure of emotional distress in private gynecologic practice, Obstet. Gynecol. 38: 139–146, 1971.
11. Rickels, K., Hesbacher, P., Fisher, E., Perloff, M. M., and Rosenfeld, H.: Emotional symptomatology in obese patients treated with fenfluramine and dextroamphetamine. In press, Psychol. Med.
12. Roth, T., Kramer, M., and Schwartz, J.: Triazolam: A sleep laboratory study of a new benzodiazepine hypnotic, Curr. Ther. Res. 16: 117–123, 1974.
13. Schwartz, J. L., Kramer, M., and Roth, T.: Triazolam: A new benzodiazepine hypnotic and its effect on mood, Curr. Ther. Res. 16: 964–970, 1974.
14. Urbach, K. F.: Hypnotic properties of amitriptyline: Comparison with secobarbital, Anesth. Analg. (Cleve.) 46: 835–842, 1967.
15. Wang, R., and Stockdale, S.: The hypnotic efficacy of triazolam, J. Int. Med. Res. 1: 600–607, 1973.
16. Zimmerman, A. M.: Comparative effects of flurazepam hydrochloride (Dalmane) and placebo in patients with insomnia, Curr. Ther. Res. 13: 18–22, 1971.

Index

Abnormal sleep: after sleeping pills, 148
Absorption: of drugs, 15, 16, 18
Abuse, potential, 17. *See also* Drug abuse
Accidents, 145; auto, 147; and insomnia, 151–52; and sleeping pills, 148*n*
Acetaldehyde, 15
Acetic acid, 15
Acetylcholine: and sleep, 48
Active sleep, 40. *See also* D-sleep
Addiction: mechanisms of, 145
Adverse reactions, 13, 15, 17, 18; to medication, 19, 21
Age: and use of sleeping pills, 28
Aggressive impulses: and insomnia, 124
Agrypnia (total insomnia), 122, 127–30
Alcohol, 9, 67, 71; and sleep, 125, 142; and sleeping pills, 21, 146*n*, 147
Alcoholic patients: sleep study in, 168
Alcohol withdrawal: treatment of, 16
Alkaloide, 10
Allergic reactions, 68, 146
Alpha chloralase, 95
Alpha-methyl-paratyrosine, 159
Alpha waves (on EEG), 37
American Cancer Society: statistics of, 149
Amino acids, 173; and sleep, 170
Amitriptyline: its effects on sleep, 124, 206–28
Amobarbital, 27, 74–76, 82, 83
Amphetamines: and sleep, 120
Amygdala: and drug action, 20
Anabolism: during sleep, 53, 54
Anal-compulsive elements, 135
Analgesic drugs, 67
Ancient Egypt, 1
Ancient Greece, 1, 6, 7
Anesthetics, 3, 59, 68

Angina pectoris, 57
Animals: sleep in, 40–42
Anteater: unusual sleep in, 41
Antianxiety agents, 20
Anticancer drugs, 143
Anticonvulsant medication, 18
Antidepressant medication, 2, 179, 206–28
Antidepressants and insomnia, 124, 125
Antihistamines, 21–22, 65–66, 97
Antipsychotic drugs, 2, 159, 179, 229–49
Anxiety: and insomnia, 113, 117, 124; about "letting go," 124; and sleep, 115–16
Apes: sleep in, 41
Apnea. *See* Sleep apnea
Arabian Nights, The, 9
ARAS. *See* Ascending reticular activating system
Aretaeus of Cappadocia, 6
Arousal: and dopamine, 48
Arousal threshold, 34, 40
Arctic circle: and sleep, 51
Ascending reticular activating system (ARAS), 44, 159; and insomnia, 120
Asclepius, 1
Association for the Psychophysiological Study of Sleep (APSS), 72
Atropine, 10
Attention: and norepinephrine, 48
Attention processes: and sleep, 53–54
Avicenna, 9
Azmitio, E., 163

Baekeland, F., 111, 128
Balter, M., 30
Barbital, 156. *See also* Barbiturates
Barbiturates: 3, 11, 12, 13–15, 28, 30, 64, 68, 74–83, 145, 152;